The American Dream *in* Tennessee:

STORIES OF FAITH, STRUGGLE, AND SURVIVAL

by

MANNY SETHI, M.D.

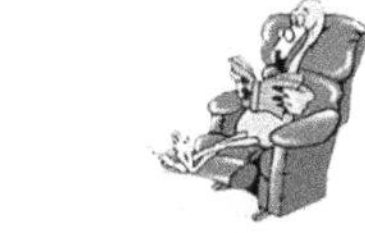

Casa Flamingo Literary Arts LLC
Nashville, TN

This book is dedicated to my parents
Dr. Brahm D. Sethi (1941-2003)
and Dr. Chander M. Sethi.
Without the sacrifices they made for
my future I would not be here today.

– MKS

The American Dream in Tennessee: Stories of Faith, Struggle, and Survival

Published by Casa Flamingo Literary Arts, Nashville, TN

www.casaflamingo.com

Hardcover first printing 2015, Softcover second printing 2017

ISBN: 978-0-9967504-0-0

Library of Congress Control Number: 2015950593

Ebook ISBN: 978-0-9743324-9-9

Cover, Page and Text Design: Jennifer Wright

Production Director: Tim O'Brien

Distribution: Ingram Global Publisher Service

TABLE OF CONTENTS

FOREWORD

In *The American Dream in Tennessee: Stories of Faith, Struggle, and Survival,* Dr. Sethi shares his story of growing up in a small town in Tennessee and his family's pursuit of the American Dream. He uses his own story and experience to set the stage for the inspiring tales of eight amazing patients who came back from near life ending trauma to resume normal lives.

While each individual life and story is unique, Dr. Sethi shows us the imperative similarities, which is the lesson of this book: Success in overcoming obstacles is never accomplished alone. It takes faith, family, and the strength of the community. As a Cardiac Transplant surgeon who was confronted with life and death situations on a daily basis, I can attest first hand to the impact of these factors in any patient's life.

As Manny did after his surgical training, I returned home in order to make a difference in the lives of patients across Tennessee. Our state is a very special place, and in each chapter of this book, one can see the unique ability of Tennesseans to reach out to one another in times of need and to make a difference.

Senator Bill Frist, M.D.
June 2015

INTRODUCTION

As an Orthopedic Trauma surgeon at Vanderbilt University Medical Center, I have been blessed to care for people across Tennessee who have been the victims of high-energy trauma. I have fought together alongside my patients as many of them stood on death's door step facing seemingly insurmountable challenges – but somehow recovered and triumphed to live a full and complete life.

Over the past three years I have spent a great deal of time with eight of these individuals exploring with them the critical factors in their road to recovery and why they were able to beat the odds. Indeed their stories are different as you will see, but the ingredients of recovery and healing are very much the same: faith, family, and the power of the community.

I have always felt a very deep kinship with my trauma patients but could honestly never put my finger on the exact reason until now. As my patients in this book opened their hearts to me and told me of their life stories and the struggle to find meaning in the midst of tragedy through their faith in God, the love of their family, and the support of the local community, I came to realize that the same factors that lead to their recovery were vital in my own life and pursuit of The American Dream in Tennessee.

Dr. Manny Sethi
August 2015

Manny

Of course I wasn't there, but I have imagined it so many times. It was a cold, foggy, winter night in New Delhi, India in the early 1970s. My father and mother were traveling in a car with my grandparents, uncles, and aunts. They had one single suitcase with all of their belongings in tow. What was running through my parents' minds as they hugged their family saying their last goodbyes? Did my dad realize it was one of the last times he would see his own father? They were leaving everything they knew behind, searching for a better life for their unborn children. Were they scared? As the plane took off in the darkness of the night could they ever imagine the future into which they were stepping?

My parents were born and raised in India and came from modest backgrounds. My father's family owned a trucking company – but during the partition they lost everything when the company and all of its trucks were burned to the ground by radicals. He, along with his siblings and parents moved to the slums of New Delhi where they were forced to start over. My mother came from a very modest family as well. My grandmother was a midwife and worked incredibly hard to support the family, as her husband was absent most of the time. After the partition, my mother also moved often with her family until they finally settled in New Delhi.

Like hundreds of other families disrupted by partition, both families basically had to make a fresh start. Moving to one of the poorest neighborhoods of New Delhi, they were determined to survive. My father, always having the deepest desire to serve humanity, chose to study medicine. The odds for him were next to impossible, but through working menial jobs and taking numerous loans he was able to put himself through medical school. I remember seeing the small room with concrete floors and walls where he would study. A single lamp and wooden desk were the sole contents. My mother also wanted to be a doctor and was clever enough to find a way to afford medical school. She served as a nanny and joined a program to work in underserved villages across India. In return, the Indian government subsidized her medical education.

She would often tell me stories of the villages in which she worked – places with no electricity or running water. She dearly missed her family, but knew this was the only way she could pay for her medical training.

My parents, both of whom shared a love of medicine and serving humanity, met through family introductions. From day one, they were completely devoted to one another and that would never change. They both greatly wanted to start a family, but my father didn't want his children to struggle like he had – to suffer the shackles of poverty and to fight for even the most basic opportunities. He also felt the acute need and responsibility to support his seven siblings who had not been able to combat poverty and abject living conditions and rise beyond it all as he had done. While growing up, he had heard much about America and the American Dream. One of his closest friends had moved to the United States and gained a great deal of success and my dad wanted that kind of opportunity for his future family.

After completing their medical training in India, my parents moved to England, where, because of their foreign medical credentials, they had to complete additional training. My older brother was born there, during a difficult time in their lives when they were house staff members, which meant they were underpaid and overworked (the equivalent of medical residency here). Often my father told me stories of how he would sleep in the back of his car between shifts. The years in England were challenging, but my parents saw England as a gateway to the United States. England didn't offer the promise of a better life, but America did.

After several years in England, my parents were ready to make the move that they had originally contemplated on that long-ago day when they left Delhi and said good bye to their families. In 1975, my parents arrived in Cleveland, Ohio with my brother (then two) in tow and a few pieces of luggage. Due to the restrictions on foreign medical graduates, my parents again had to go through additional training in order to become licensed physicians in this country. That meant years of additional hard work; but it did not deter either of them. For the future of their children and the pursuit of the American Dream they so desperately sought, they did residency again, for the third time!

In Ohio, my parents and brother settled into a dingy one bedroom apartment in a run-down part of Cleveland, which was the best they could afford. I was born two years later, in the middle of what was one of the worst blizzards Cleveland had ever seen. As resident physicians they made very little money and making ends meet with two young children was hard, but they did it. On their few days off they would work extra overnight shifts to make money. After they finished residency, we moved to Chicago for a short time and finally to Hillsboro, Tennessee in 1983, a small town outside Manchester, just south of Nashville. They were two of the first physicians in the area. Dad was a primary care doctor and mom was an OBGYN who at one time in that town's history had delivered half of its babies!

As a five-year-old I vividly remember the excitement of seeing our new home for the first time. We had always lived in small one or two bedroom apartments in run-down neighborhoods, but this was clearly different – a brick house with a yard and trees! Growing up in Hillsboro was an incredible experience. From the get-go, our neighbors took a deep interest in our lives and I learned so much from all my new friends. Our home was next to a large farm so I spent many of my days exploring and playing in the cornfields with other kids from my neighborhood. My parents enrolled me in Little League and I developed a deep passion for baseball. I will never forget one of the games when I was in fourth grade playing for C and H Construction. (Many years later, in the emergency room, I would operate on my first coach who had sustained a terrible fall).

It was my first game. I had been up to bat two times and had struck out both times. It was my third try and everyone could tell I was scared. Suddenly from the stands I could hear our neighbors and friends shouting words of encouragement, "You can do it Tony, come on." Everyone on the team had a nickname and mine was Tony, the name my brother chose out of his love for Tony the Tiger, the mascot on the cover of Kellogg's Frosted Flakes cereal. I will never forget that Saturday morning in Fred Deadman Park. On my next swing I hit a home run. The encouragement and love in that moment was very potent. I was learning the power of community.

Hillsboro was a strong community. Along with my mom and dad, our neighbors and friends had a strong hand in raising my brother and me, teaching us values as we grew. If I misbehaved at the city pool or said a curse word on the field, you can bet that mom and dad would know about it even before I got home. Neighbors were always there for one another and you could count on them to reach out in times of need. Hillsboro was a farming community and people didn't have much money, but we always had each other. I remember many of my friends in elementary school were happy to be in school just so they could have the two meals served every day. While spending time with my friends after school or during sleep overs, I realized how hard it was for the farming community to make ends meet and the incredible amount of work it took.

My mom and dad quickly became pillars within the community. Being the only doctors in town in the early 1980s, they got to know everyone. In many cases they treated an entire family and served as doctor, psychologist, and occasionally even the marriage counselor! Every Sunday when we would go grocery shopping I remember all the proud mothers showing my mom the beautiful babies she had delivered, and as the years went by the babies of those babies. Back in the early 1980s there weren't many ambulances available, so frequently I would travel around the back roads of Coffee County with my dad as he visited sick patients. It wasn't unusual for us to take some of my dad's patients to the hospital when they were too sick to be cared for at home.

Outside of my family, one person who had a tremendous influence on my upbringing was Billy-Joe Weitz, the maintenance man for our local hospital who ultimately worked for my parents helping out around their medical clinic. When I was a kid, my parents were very busy caring for their patients. My mother would often leave in the middle of the night to deliver babies and my dad was constantly in the clinic or on-call in the Manchester Hospital emergency room. Billy-Joe started out helping my parents in the clinic, but as mom and dad grew to know and trust him, he became an all-around family helper. Whether it was picking me up from school, taking me to baseball practice, or cheering me on at a basketball game, Billy-Joe and I spent many hours together.

Many of my best memories include sitting in the passenger seat of his beat-up blue Ford truck listening to country music radio through the one speaker that worked. To this day, whenever I hear singers like the Judds or Randy Travis, I can't help but be transported back to Billy-Joe's blue truck.

I confided in Billy-Joe on nearly everything. Looking back, I learned so much from him about hard work and Tennessee values. Win or lose, good day or bad day, when I was in that truck listening to country music, my problems melted away and I would slowly start to feel better about whatever was bugging me. However, Billy-Joe was no push over, and often I was his assistant maintenance man. My parents from the start wanted me to understand the value of a dollar and made it clear to Billy-Joe that I would have to carry my own weight, so on weekends and after school, he made me work, whether it was mowing two acres of grass, buffing floors, or painting walls.

While growing up, some of my best times were in the gym, playgrounds, and classrooms of Hillsboro Elementary School. Spending seven years there, I got to know every inch of the school and made lasting friendships. But then as my friends moved to Manchester Junior High, I received a big surprise – my parents wanted to send me to The Webb School, a private academy in nearby Bell Buckle. Leaving my friends in the fall of 1989 for a new school was daunting, but I quickly came to love Webb and the little village. With a population of less than five-hundred folks, Bell Buckle was similar to Hillsboro in that everyone knew everyone.

Honor and faith were two fundamental principals at Webb. On every test we would write a pledge that we did not cheat and our word was our bond. Faith was a big part of the Webb experience: every morning in Chapel we would sing hymns like Amazing Grace (which still remains my favorite hymn) and read different passages from the Bible. I will never forget one of our teachers who would always preach about the willingness to continue forward in the face of adversity; he would read John 11:43. Even today when I face situations that seem insurmountable, I think of the story of Lazarus, who rose from the ashes four days after his death.

As I grew older, I started noticing problems with my dad's health. Starting when I was in middle school, in 1991, he was in and out of clinics seeing specialists and was admitted to the hospital many times to undergo major blood transfusions. I remember at one point he looked so frail that we were all worried he wouldn't make it. He was eventually diagnosed with an autoimmune disorder known as Sarcoidosis, which is a rare disorder that attacked every organ in his body. I will never forget the nights I stayed by his side at the hospital. Even lying in a hospital bed getting a blood transfusion, he had such strength and courage that he would reassure me, "listen, go study. Things will be fine, I didn't come this far to leave you now." It was at these times as a young boy that I turned to faith. I didn't know what else to do but to pray that things would be okay. Ultimately with a lot of help from doctors and the support of my mother, dad got back on his feet and started practicing medicine again. He deeply cared for the people of Hillsboro and Manchester and felt a profound responsibility to continue providing for his family.

During the next few years his health improved and we returned to life as normal. High school went by so fast, and I made so many life-long friends and met the love of my life, Maya. We were both seventeen and attending summer school in Boston the summer before we became high school seniors in 1995. It was literally love at first sight and I knew she was the one for me. She was from a small town in Ohio just outside Cleveland. On the bank of the Charles River one day, I asked her to be my girlfriend and from that moment on we were soul mates. I fell madly in love with her. Every day after summer classes let out, we would spend time together and after that summer was over we wrote each other letters every day – nearly a decade later we would get married.

Throughout high school I was torn on the direction of my future. I had grown up around my parents' clinic seeing the power of medicine and its abilities to forge relationships in the community, and I had seen my mom and dad save many lives. But at the same time I felt the need to do something different. That is, until I worked for Senator Bill Frist the summer after graduating from high school. Interning with the senator was a life-changing experience. He was the kind of guy who took you under his wing and wanted to help guide you through life. He repeatedly told me about his experiences as a surgeon and how amazing it was to have the ability to save lives. I will never forget the walk I took with him to the top of the Capitol Rotunda in Washington, D.C. on my last day working for him. We had walked for nearly an hour when he asked me what I wanted to do with my life. He assured me that no matter what I did, as long as it was centered on service to humanity, I would be successful. After that summer, I knew I would become a surgeon.

After graduating from Webb in 1996 and spending that summer with the senator, I began the long journey to become a surgeon, a journey that in many ways began in my parents' clinic in Manchester and in Bill Frist's office. I went to college at Brown University in Rhode Island where I was a premedical student. During those years my relationship with Maya, who was a student at Wellesley College, continued to blossom. We would spend virtually every weekend studying together in the library and working toward the future. But as I finished college I felt this yearning to do something much greater than myself – to give back and to see the world.

Upon graduation from Brown in 2000, and through the support of the Fulbright Fellowship, a State Department funded program designed to create meaningful bonds between American college graduates and foreign countries, I represented the United States in Tunisia, a small country in North Africa. Tunisia has a high prevalence of Limb Girdle Muscular Dystrophy, a genetic degenerative disease of the muscle. Affected families are often impoverished and geographically isolated; many children never receive treatment and die at an early age. For one year after college, I worked with a team of medical professionals helping Tunisian children and their families gain access to healthcare and cope with muscular dystrophy. We traveled the country and started to build a national registry of afflicted children that was ultimately used to coordinate care, and conducted research that investigated the genetic basis of the disease. Families often sought us out as a central access point, seeking counseling and connections with local neurologists.

In Tunisia, I saw much poverty and suffering, but I also witnessed the power of medicine and compassion that built lasting bridges. I will never forget children like Amal and the conversations I had with her family. I had never imagined explaining to Bedouin parents the devastating impact that Limb Girdle Muscular Dystrophy would have on their daughter. In Arabic, "Amal" means "hope" and we reached out to the Tunisian community to provide it. It was incredibly painful to explain to Amal's parents that her difficulty with walking was due to a disease that would never leave her, and she would require a wheelchair for the rest of her life. But because of our work, my colleagues and I were also able to connect Amal and her family with medical specialists and other resources that would not have otherwise been available to them. My experiences with children like Amal and their families demonstrated to me the powerful relationships that evolve through a commitment to global community service. My experiences also further strengthened my resolve to become a physician.

After my year in Tunisia, I pursued medical school at Harvard while Maya began law school at Vanderbilt University in Nashville, where she was able to spend more time with my family. She would spend weekends in Hillsboro and then tell me about all the wonderful things that were going on with my family that I missed. But the days went by quickly and I loved learning the art of medicine. I would attend classes or be in the hospital all day and study in the libraries most of the night. While I missed the love of my life and being at home in Tennessee, I was enthralled with the workings of the human body.

That is, until my world collapsed around me. I will never forget that hot summer day in the middle of August 2003, right before I was about to start my second year of medical school. As I was walking home from the hospital, my mother called and I immediately knew something was wrong. "Sit down," she said. I quickly found a bench near a park where some young kids were playing soccer and as I sat and watched the kids, I listened to my mother tell me that my father had nearly passed out at work and was taken to the hospital. The lab work had shown some major abnormalities and the doctors could feel a large mass in his liver.

"He is going to Nashville tomorrow for more tests," my mother said. I immediately felt weak in my knees, almost paralyzed. It was surreal watching the children play soccer without a care in the world while I sat there and faced the fact that something was very wrong with my father.

The next morning I flew to Nashville on the first flight out and met my parents at St. Thomas Hospital. As my dad got the CT scan I stood in front of the monitor watching the results. As the scanner showed his liver, a wave of nausea came over me; there were tumors everywhere. I saw my mother from the corner of my eye, who hadn't seen the CT scan yet. "How am I going to tell her?" I wondered. I will never forget later that day as I stood in the baggage claim of Nashville airport waiting to pick up my brother who had by this time become a surgeon – he took one look at me and knew exactly what I was going to say.

The following months were a struggle. The doctor told us my dad had three months to live so I took a leave of absence from medical school and moved home to help take care of him. Every day he told me to go back to medical school and complete his mission of coming to America by becoming a doctor, but I wanted to stay with him. In the final days of his life he fought valiantly, never wanting to show others the pain he felt. Rather, he would talk to me about the future and about my plans. He deeply loved Maya and wanted me to marry her and implored me to take care of my mother when he was gone. I would watch as person after person, patient after patient, would come to our small home to say their goodbyes. He always tried to comfort them, to leave them with something uplifting. He fought until the end and on Oct. 27, 2003, he died in the very hospital in Manchester that he had helped survive for so many years. I was twenty-four years old without a father, and I was numb with pain but within two weeks I returned to medical school. The first day back, as I walked to the hospital at 4:30 a.m. in two feet of Boston snow, I cried in the darkness. My tears froze on my face as I kept playing his words over and over that I had to complete the mission, finish what he had started on that foggy night when he left Delhi.

The coming years were difficult as I sank into an abyss of sadness. Maya transferred from Vanderbilt to Boston University School of Law to be by my side – but I was not myself without Dad. It took everything I had to finish medical school but things weren't the same. Throughout this time my mother did her best to support and stand by me. She reminded me of what she and my father wanted for my brother and I and pushed me to continue forward. Despite feeling alone without my father and overwhelmed without him, she always remained strong for the family – she is an amazing woman and would sacrifice anything for her kids. "I believe in you," she would repeatedly tell me.

I had no choice but to stay the course. I knew what my dad would have wanted me to do. Thinking about what Senator Frist had told me so many years before, at the end of medical school, I chose to pursue orthopedic surgery training at Massachusetts General Hospital in Boston for the next five years. But my residency training years were grueling – both physically and mentally – and I felt increasingly disconnected from my friends and family. I was losing my sense of direction and faith. While I applied myself in the operating room and was slowly becoming a good surgeon, without my father it lost all meaning, things were different. I constantly questioned my path and my relationship with Maya, by now my wife, started to become turbulent. It was almost like being in quick sand; no matter what I did I just felt like it was hard to stay afloat. I continued to blame myself for what had happened to my father, that I had not been there enough, that I could and should have diagnosed his illness during its early stages.

But when I least expected it, God reached out his hand. I was in Los Angeles with Maya at a friend's wedding, and things couldn't have been worse. I was exhausted and angry with little hope. My passion for surgery and medicine had dried up to an all time low, my future was unclear, and there I was flipping the channels of the television. Suddenly I came upon Joel Osteen, the famous pastor at Lakewood Church in Houston, Texas, delivering a televised sermon. I have no idea to this day why my remote control stopped there as it did. He quoted from Corinthians about dealing with loss, about hope and about faith. He talked about holding onto God and holding onto faith when there is nothing else to hold onto, about believing in one's self and how everyone has a purpose.

The pastor's words stuck with me the entire weekend and gave me a sense of hope and optimism I hadn't felt in a long time; I could not stop thinking about his sermon. Maya and I started to watch his sermons each week and read his books that expounded upon the power of living a positive and faith filled life. I started to take stock of what was happening around me. I realized I had come to a low point in my life and that I had to turn things around. I had to find my passion again that had once so powerfully driven me forward. I started once again to read the Bible that was given to me upon my graduation from Webb. I found myself thinking a great deal about Hillsboro and the people who had made such a difference in my life. I started to realize that my purpose, my mission in life, was going to be dedicated to help the people who had helped our family. I wanted to return home to Tennessee.

For so long, because of my sadness, I had shut out many of my life-long friends. Seeing them again reminded me of dad. But I realized that these were the very people who I needed; the people who could help me heal, folks who really cared about me. I started to reach out once again to my childhood friends and to find my way back home. I will never forget one of my visits back to Manchester; I was in Evelyn's Office Supplies store when the owner showed me her hand which had a large scar. She then proceeded to tell me how she had been in a car accident and how my dad had saved her life. My father was gone, but right before me was a hand he stitched and a life he had saved.

From that moment forward, I started to regain a sense of who I was and why I had pursued my own particular path. I developed a deep interest in trauma surgery and started to hone my skills. Maya and I refocused on each other and became closer than ever and we started to plan our return to Tennessee. I once again reached out to Dr. Bill Frist who was now teaching at Princeton University. After so many years, as any great mentor does, he took the time to guide me. For more than an hour on the phone, he quietly listened and encouraged me to return to Tennessee and suggested I work in the trauma department at Vanderbilt University. The next day I learned that Dr. Frist had already arranged an interview at Vanderbilt University Medical Center for me.

In 2010 Maya and I came back home. It was always hard flying back into Nashville; I would think of my dad standing at the gate waiting for me and giving me a hug. It was an incredible feeling to be home; to know I was here to stay. But my first year at Vanderbilt as an orthopedic trauma fellow turned out to be the most challenging of my surgical training. Working eighteen hour days that started at 4:30 a.m., I saw trauma like I had never seen it before, because Vanderbilt is one of the few Level 1 Trauma Centers across three states and receives a huge volume of trauma. My mentor at Vanderbilt was a man by the name of Bill Obremskey, an incredible surgeon. He taught me how to think critically in chaotic situations and to always make choices that put the patient first. He had an incredible story himself. After being infected with a flesh eating bacteria and spending weeks in an intensive care unit where he almost died, he fought his way back to the operating room. Of everyone I met, Dr. Obremskey was the only one who filled part of the void inside me and helped guide me in the right direction. I still look up to him, and thank him, today.

After finishing my training, I was fortunate enough to receive an offer of permanent employment to stay at Vanderbilt. Every day I thank God for the tremendous privilege I have to take care of victims of trauma and be a part of their lives, their families, and their recovery. These people are good, hard-working Tennesseans who had the misfortune of being critically injured on the job or from just simple, everyday life and chores. Many of them remind me of the good folks of Hillsboro who had a hand in raising me. No matter the adversity, they march onward and always try to stay positive. I remember one day as I wheeled a patient into surgery, he asked me to pray with him. Afterward, he looked at me and revealed, "I knew you when you were this small," as he held his hand about three feet from the ground. Injured badly in a car accident, the man told me how he had once been a patient of my father and how my mother had delivered his two sons. In moments like this I felt God was talking directly to me, telling me that this was my place and my purpose.

In addition to working at Vanderbilt University Medical Center, I began developing a practice at Nashville General Hospital and Meharry Medical College. Meharry was the county hospital, and I was shocked at the level of poverty and suffering I saw in many of my patients. Many of these folks had nowhere to turn, and I was privileged to become their surgeon and doctor. While working at Meharry, I started to see a great deal of youth violence – shootings, stabbings, and beatings. Many of my patients were victims of violence and didn't trust me from the onset. I did my best to form relationships with them, to show them that I cared and to implore them to change the direction of their life before a fatal injury happened.

One patient I will never forget was a young man who was the victim of a particularly bad stabbing. He started to curse at me when we first met and told me that I didn't care about him. But one month later, after many visits to my clinic where I worked hard to save his leg, he began to trust me. All he needed to see was that I truly was invested in his life and his future. In these moments, I began to grasp the power of compassion and understanding to build bridges.

In working with impoverished children and young adults, I realized that the vast majority of these kids were good people but that the conflicts they were involved with got out of hand very quickly because they didn't have the skills to control and stop the situation. I grew increasingly concerned and frustrated with treating such young trauma victims. Ultimately, my experiences treating these young trauma victims led me to develop a simple conflict resolution program for middle school children that I introduced to schools across Nashville and later Memphis. The basis of the program is that if kids can learn conflict resolution skills on the front end in school, we could potentially avoid seeing them as victims of violence in the emergency rooms. I have deeply appreciated partnering with teachers and school leaders across the city to implement the conflict resolution program. My time in Metro Nashville Public Schools and Memphis schools has reminded me so much of my positive experiences with teachers at Hillsboro Elementary and Webb School who did so much to shape me.

While work kept me busy, Maya remained the center of my life. She has always been very understanding and supportive of the life of a trauma surgeon and my drive to do something for our community. We had talked so much about having a family and finally were ready. After much struggle that led us to many doctors and lots of praying, we had our miracle baby in June 2013. I will never forget the first night bringing J.B. home and putting him to bed. I cried tears of joy for the gift that God had given us and prayed that I would be the best father and husband I could be.

After having little J.B., I started to think more and more about the future. Being a doctor and seeing patients from across the state, I was acutely aware that many of our citizens were not healthy and that costs of care were rising dramatically. Watching our state's Medicaid program "Tenn Care" take more than thirty percent of our state budget, I started to visit state legislators to talk with them about what we could do to improve healthcare and reduce costs. Most of the time I watched eyes glaze over as I talked to state leaders – they appeared to care less. One legislator actually said to me, "The only way you will make any difference is by writing me a check." Night after night talking to Maya she finally said, "Well, you should do something about this if it gets you so frustrated."

Out of this discussion came Healthy Tennessee, a non-profit Maya and I created to focus on preventative care and healthy lifestyles. Through Healthy Tennessee we started to hold health fairs and lectures across the state, talking to people about healthy lifestyles. I deeply enjoyed my travels across Tennessee, remembering the places my dad had taken me when I was a boy and meeting so many people with powerful stories. At one fair we met a small girl who had not seen out of one eye for many years but had never seen an ophthalmologist. We connected her with the right doctors and she was diagnosed with glaucoma and successfully cured. At another health fair I examined a gentleman who had a blood pressure of 200/110, twice what it should be and certain to cause damage to his internal organs. I asked him why he had not received care and he told me the story of how he had lost his trucking job and health insurance. Together we thought about ways he could improve his blood pressure through diet and exercise and I will never forget what he said. "Right now it's my problem, but at some point, it will be somebody else's problem." We could treat his high blood pressure for 10 cents daily. Once the high pressures damaged his kidney and liver, a likely scenario, that price could rise to $100,000 per day. As I traveled Tennessee, I came to realize that stories like this take place every day.

Whether it was working with children teaching them ways to avoid violence or talking to folks about healthy lifestyles, the one thing I came to love was that power of the community, the power that I first felt growing up in Hillsboro. Whether it is in Sparta, Milan, or Johnson City, Tennesseans really care about one another and have the will and desire to work together to make things better for themselves and their communities.

Ultimately, that is what this book is really about – the power of faith, community, and family to help each of us overcome challenge and move forward. I often think about my mother and father getting on that airplane in New Delhi without a clue of what the future would be, but knowing they wanted a better future for their unborn children. Without their courageous act and the loving arms of the Hillsboro community, I would never have lived the life I have. When tragedy struck my family and we lost Dad it was the power of faith that helped me overcome the darkest period of my life. Faith gave me the power to fight onward and helped me to see my ultimate mission – to return home and improve the lives of those who had made my American Dream in Tennessee a reality.

In the springtime of hope, faith remains eternal, my spirit remains strong, and my father's light for a better tomorrow remains as brilliant as the day he left India for not only me, but ultimately for the victims of trauma who I have been blessed to come into contact with in the operating room. Every sunrise is a testament for God's love for us, and every sunset reminds me of a day long ago when my father began a voyage for our family that continues on. I eagerly await the next chapter that God has prepared.

In the following chapters I share eight powerful stories of my patients, all victims of near life-ending trauma, who overcame incredible odds to survive. While the names of my patients and their loved ones have been changed to protect identities, their stories are all true. Through their faith in God, and support of their families and the love of their communities, these individuals came back from severe injuries to move forward in their lives. In each story the power of Tennesseans to overcome adversity and triumph in the face of great challenge is clear. Incredibly, our stories are intertwined in many ways. The power of faith and the love of community and family that made me who I am and has allowed me to live the American Dream is the same foundation which healed these individuals.

Aaron

Much like me, Aaron is a Tennessee boy. He grew up in Nashville and found his love for music one decade before he found God. Following in the footsteps of his older brothers, Lucas and Ethan, Aaron picked up his first bass guitar when he was fourteen years old. After their parents divorced, his brothers moved to California to live with their father. They had created their own band and wanted to make it big in the music industry. The younger Aaron remained in Nashville with his mother, but he longed to be in his brothers' band. Still, he knew there was no better place to learn musical skills than right at home in Music City.

Aaron's friend Ben played guitar and the two of them enjoyed playing music together. A couple other boys from school joined their band and before they were old enough to be admitted as customers to the clubs on Nashville's Lower Broadway, the local music scene, Aaron and his friends were booking gigs at the clubs.

Within a few years, Aaron's brothers returned to Nashville and when they heard Aaron play for the first time, they invited him to join their band. Aaron was thrilled. In honor of their brotherhood, they changed the name of their heavy rock metal band to Matthews.

The three brothers began playing gigs around the city, joining hundreds of other young Nashville musicians in their chase for the elusive record deal. Music was their passion, but the temptations that came with a rock music life were too sweet to pass up. Aaron began drinking and experimenting with drugs. The high that he felt rocking out on stage under the influence of marijuana and alcohol was exhilarating.

When he was still eighteen, Aaron found out his high school sweetheart, Sheryl, was pregnant. As the son of divorced parents, Aaron was determined to make it work with Sheryl and they got married before she gave birth to their daughter, Maria. At the same time, his brother Lucas joined a traveling band and Aaron and the Matthews broke up.

To support his family, Aaron started working at a woodshop making cabinets. He made a decent living for a few years and he worked hard, but the nine-to-five life wasn't for him. He missed the thrill of performing and the out-of-body euphoria that he experienced while under the influence of drugs. He reasoned if he couldn't play music for a living like his brother Lucas, he wanted to be surrounded by those who did. He began working for a company that built road cases, an instrument case that bands use when they tour. For the next several years, Aaron continued working there, but he was still very much dependent on drugs and alcohol, and his life began to take a downward spiral.

Aaron knew something had to change and deep down he had a feeling that Jesus was the answer. He didn't know much about God and religion. When he was much younger, his grandparents would show him pictures of Jesus and he would hear them pray and hold Bible studies together. Now as an adult, Aaron had no idea who Jesus was, but he felt that if he did, his life might improve.

Tyler, one of Aaron's co-workers, was a devout Christian and he could be seen praying several times throughout the day. Aaron had never talked to Tyler about his faith but he wondered what it was like to have a relationship with God. He wanted to talk with Tyler about God but he couldn't gather up the nerve to ask. It was like a large elephant in the room that both of them pretended not to notice, knowing fully well that the other person was aware of its presence.

One day, while they were getting ready to leave work, Tyler walked up to Aaron and asked, quite bluntly, "Aaron, do you believe in God?"

Aaron was caught off guard. "I don't know," he responded truthfully.

"Where do you think you will go when you die?" asked Tyler.

"I don't know," repeated Aaron, feeling uneasy. "You're getting all deep on me."

Aaron walked away from Tyler and headed for home.

For the next few weeks, Aaron did everything he could to avoid Tyler's interrogation about his faith. Still, Tyler remained persistent.

"I'm serious man," said Tyler, with urgency in voice. "If you were going to die today, right this second, where are you going?"

Aaron paused in thought and the last decade of his life flashed before his eyes. "I don't know," he said quietly. They both stood in silence. Finally, Aaron admitted, "I hope I'd go to heaven."

"Do you want to find out?" asked Tyler. "Are you interested in learning about God and Jesus?"

"I am," said Aaron.

Tyler led Aaron out to his truck. Tyler taught Aaron a prayer, and the two of them began praying. After a short time, Tyler turned to Aaron and said, "You have accepted Jesus in your heart. You are saved."

Aaron had no idea what that meant. "What do I do now?" asked Aaron.

"Go home and start reading the Book of John, it's written for new believers like you and describes the death and resurrection of Jesus. Pray that God will reveal himself to you through his word." He handed Aaron a Bible.

For the next few weeks, Aaron became absorbed in the Bible. He had a gut feeling, like something was tugging at him. He still wasn't sure he believed in God, but when he got this feeling, he felt he was being led in the right direction.

During this same time David, another friend, invited Aaron and Sheryl to join him at church in south Nashville. It was a Lutheran church, and they joined him for a Sunday service. As the pastor shared his sermon, Aaron looked around at the other church members. Most of them sat back in the pews, appearing to have dozed off. Aaron whispered to Sheryl, "I don't think this is for me."

The next Sunday Tyler and Aaron went to another church in Clarksville, a small city fifty miles north of Nashville. When the service began, Aaron watched in awe as the congregation stood around him, shouting, singing and praising God. It was as if he were at a concert. Aaron felt that familiar internal tugging and knew he had found a spiritual home.

Life at home with Sheryl was tough. She didn't support his new found love for God. She also used drugs and alcohol and wanted him to continue to do so as well and he couldn't help but give in when she used. A part of him wondered if anything or anyone was powerful enough to break this addiction.

Aaron continued reading his Bible. He read the Book of John and the Four Gospels, and learned of the Holy Spirit. He had heard of the Holy Spirit before but had no idea about His power. Aaron became even more intrigued and decided to talk about it with Tyler.

Tyler laughed when Aaron brought up the Holy Spirit to him over lunch one day. "Oh man, I don't know if you want to go there."

The more Aaron read about the Baptism in the Holy Spirit, he became more and more fascinated with the idea of it. He read about worshippers speaking in tongues and having the supernatural power of God flowing through them. He wanted to find that passion, that exhilaration within religion and his faith. If God was real, then Aaron needed to experience the Baptism of the Holy Spirit to truly believe.

Tyler and Aaron went back to the Assemblies of God's church in Clarksville. It was a Wednesday night, and the service was quiet and dead. It didn't seem like the Holy Spirit was flowing at all within the church. As the pastor gave his sermon, Aaron waited anxiously and after what seemed like centuries, the preacher announced the altar call.

"Are you ready to leave?" Tyler asked.

"Nope," he said simply. "I came here to be filled with the Spirit, and by God I am going to get it." He stood up and approached the altar. When Aaron said he wanted to receive the baptism of the Holy Spirit, the pastor's eyes became wide with joy.

Suddenly, the service came to life. The congregation began talking excitedly and crowding around him. After taking a few minutes to read scripture, they began praying. Aaron welcomed that familiar internal tug. Everyone continued praying. Although he began quietly at first, soon Aaron began to praise the Lord aloud. After a few seconds, Aaron couldn't help but yell out his praises to God. He began chanting at the top of his lungs.

All at once a jolt of electricity shot up from Aaron's feet. It traveled up his legs, through his arms, and all the way up to his head. The immense power pulled Aaron to the floor, where he lay on his back facing the ceiling. Tongues uncontrollably began spilling out of his mouth.

This was incredible. The rush that Aaron was feeling was unlike any he had ever experienced. His mind flashed back to all the times he had abused drugs. The miniscule highs he had gotten from those substances were laughable compared to the complete exultation he was feeling in that moment. As he lay there, possessed by the Holy Spirit, he heard a small voice say, "How does this compare to your drugs and alcohol?"

Aaron lost control. He began weeping. He lay on the floor of the church, embodied by the Holy Spirit for nearly an hour. When he finally let the Holy Spirit pass from his body, everyone around him stood in complete silence.

Aaron was a see-it-to-believe-it kind of guy. Since that moment, he never lost his faith for a single second. However, Sheryl continued to tempt him with drugs, threatening to divorce him once again if he continued down a religious path. For the first time he felt like he had the strength to leave her and get a divorce. Aaron wanted a fresh start, so he decided to leave not only Sheryl, but his job at the cabinet company. But while he struggled to find a new job, the temptations of drugs were once again too strong. He began using again, this time with even harder drugs, like cocaine and LSD. Eventually, he was able to find work as an electrician for a company that made tour buses. It was a relief to not only have a new job, but it led him to Virginia. A sweet, beautiful woman, Virginia made Aaron's heart flutter. When he finally worked up the nerve to ask her out on a date, she said yes. From their first night out, he knew he wanted Virginia to be his wife.

Virginia's relationship with Aaron mirrored mine with my wife Maya. She meant everything to him and he loved her more than life itself. She understood him and changed the direction and path of his life – she made him a better person.

A few years later, Aaron experienced another miracle – his sweet Virginia was pregnant with his child. The day Aaron first put their daughter Katie in his arms, he knew God would watch over the both of them.

When Katie was a baby, she would often fall, getting scrapes and bruises. So when Katie broke her leg when she was two, Aaron didn't think much of it. A year later, when she fell and had to get stitches on her lip, Aaron knew she would heal in no time. But when Katie was three, and the doctor called Virginia and Aaron and told them that Katie had contracted a severe MRSA blood infection, Aaron's world turned upside down.

Although doctors treated her initial symptoms, the MRSA kept coming back. They said now that Katie had contracted it, she would always be susceptible to outbreaks. Aaron didn't know how to deal with seeing his daughter suffer. This time, instead of turning to God, he turned the other way.

A few months after Katie's first outbreak, Aaron sat in the park, lighting up his pipe full of marijuana. Katie had experienced another infection outbreak. Aaron and Virginia were desperate. They really thought her last outbreak would be the last time. Virginia began crying, and Aaron knew that this had to stop.

"God," he said, his voice trembling, "I can't take it anymore. I'd do anything to get this child healed. I'll go back to church. I will quit doing drugs, I promise you."

Just as He had when Aaron had asked for the Baptism of the Holy Spirit, God listened. Katie never had another break out since that day. Staying true to his end of the bargain, the grass Aaron smoked that day was his last. He had his promise to God to keep, and he began looking for a church for his family.

During the prior ten years, Aaron's brothers had recovered from drugs and alcohol and had found the Lord as well. They found a church called Highland Park Church in Nashville, where they played in the band during services. The small but mighty church held services in a high school auditorium.

When Aaron asked his brother Lucas about joining his church, Lucas was delighted. "You know, Aaron, we could really use a bass player."

It was as if God had given them a second chance. Once again, the Matthews brothers were living their passion for music together, this time for Jesus. Aaron never felt more at peace.

Everything in Aaron's life began to fall into place. He didn't get along with his boss at the coach company who would lie to his customers and then ask Aaron to cover for him. Now, as a true Christian, Aaron couldn't do it. One Sunday morning at home, he prayed for God's help in getting out of this toxic situation. Shortly thereafter, he received a phone call from one of the customers, Bobby.

"Hey Aaron, I have been praying about something. We want to start our own interior shop, and we want you to be a part of it."

During the next few months, Aaron, Alec, and a few of his friends began working in a small interior shop in Gallatin. All were devout Christians and they would begin each week with a Bible study.

A few blissful years later, Aaron and Virginia got married on Eagle Glacier in Juneau, Alaska. Life with her and their daughter was perfect. They spent several years enjoying a peaceful life in East Nashville.

Aaron loved working with his Christian brothers in the shop. He bought a motorcycle that he rode to work on days when the weather was good.

On one day in March, Aaron checked the weather as he always did before setting out on his bike. He would never chance riding if rain was in the forecast, but today promised to be a perfectly sunny day. He kissed Virginia and Katie, put on his helmet, and headed off to work.

He was working on building a bus for the Randy Rogers Band in the shop when one of his vendors, Peter, called and asked him if he wanted to have lunch at O'Charley's in Gallatin. Aaron needed to pick up a part for Nathan, one of his co-workers, so he got on his bike and headed over to the restaurant.

Aaron and Peter had lunch, but an hour later when he went to start his motorcycle to head back to work, he realized he had left the light on and the battery was dead. Aaron called Nathan, who said he would come over and help him get the bike started.

While he waited for Nathan, Aaron called Virginia at work.

"What's wrong?" Virginia said the moment she picked up. She wasn't used to Aaron calling during the middle of the day.

"Don't worry sweetie," Aaron said with a chuckle, "My bike needs to be jumped and I just wanted to call to say I love you while I waited."

"Oh sweetie, I love you too," said Virginia softly.

It remains incredible to me that Aaron made this call when he did, perhaps he knew something was going to happen? It reminds me of my final conversation with Billy-Joe, who had such a powerful impact on my up-bringing. A few days before leaving for medical school Billy-Joe came over to the house to say good-bye as he always did. But this time was different – he never became emotional but this time he began to tear up and told me how proud of me he was and how much I meant to him. One month later Billy-Joe passed away.

By the time Aaron got off the phone, Nathan had arrived and had gotten Aaron's bike started. Aaron put on his helmet and climbed on and headed back to work. As he rode down the road, with the wind in his face, he couldn't help but smile. After a few miles, he slowed down as he approached a three-way intersection.

He had two paths ahead of him. If he went left, he would go directly back to work. If he went straight, he would take the scenic way back. He decided to take the scenic route.

It was a beautiful day and he felt happy and blessed. Aaron's relationship with God had flourished under his new job, where he would read his Bible every day. A few months earlier, for their New Year's Resolution, Virginia and Aaron had decided to start tithing 10 percent of their income to the church every week. Life was good.

Aaron lifted his foot, reared up his bike, and sped off.

At that very second, a car pulled out of a side street and crashed into his motorcycle. Aaron was thrown approximately thirty feet in to the air and with a loud thud, landed on the side of the road like a broken rag doll.

Onlookers screamed with horror. Blood was everywhere. It was flowing out of gashes that covered Aaron's body and his face. His arm was twisted behind his back as if it was completely detached from his body. His right leg was nearly ripped off.

Police quickly arrived guiding a parade of paramedics behind them. One of the policemen ran out of his vehicle and rushed to Aaron, kneeling at his side. He examined Aaron's wounds. Within a few moments, he realized that this man was going to die. Still kneeling on the side of the road, he held up his hands and began to pray.

That day, another EMT named Joseph Martinez was driving by the scene when he saw what had happened. He jumped out of his car and joined the rest of the EMTs who were rushing to Aaron's aid.

Andrew Pope, one of the top EMTs in the division, was among those who had rushed to Aaron's aid. When he saw Aaron, he began giving directions and quickly the EMTs were moving Aaron to the ambulance. His right leg fell to the side, hanging on to the rest of his body by only a few pieces of flesh. One of the EMTs held Aaron's broken left arm with terror. It was like holding a wet noodle.

Aaron was as pale as a ghost. He was losing blood quickly and they felt that he would be dead by the time they arrived at Vanderbilt Hospital.

"He won't make it," said Andrew. "We need to stop at Sumner County and get him stabilized."

The ambulance sped off. When they got to the Sumner Regional Medical Center they began giving Aaron blood. It took eighteen pints before he was stabilized enough to move him to Vanderbilt.

As Aaron was being rushed to Vanderbilt, Virginia was just leaving work, the sweet sound of Aaron's voice still ringing in her ear. She picked up Katie from daycare and the two of them went home. Usually Aaron called her on her ride home but by the time they arrived at the house that day, Virginia hadn't received that phone call.

She got home, put down her purse, leaned back in her recliner, and began opening up the mail. Within seconds, there was a knock on the door. She got up, opened the door and standing before her was a policeman.

"Virginia Matthews?" he asked breathlessly.

"Yes?" She said, her forehead wrinkled in confusion.

Everything after that moment was a blur. She heard him say Aaron, motorcycle, and wreck.

"Katie!" she screamed. "Come downstairs, we have to go!"

Virginia and her daughter climbed into the back of the police car headed off to Vanderbilt. She recalls that it seemed like the policeman was going 100 miles per hour, his sirens blaring. Still, it was the longest trip of her life. The first person she called was her stepfather, who was a pastor. The second was Aaron's co-worker Alec. He explained that Aaron had not come back from lunch two hours earlier. He was shocked when he heard Virginia tell him what happened.

When they arrived at Vanderbilt's Emergency Room, Virginia was rushed to the side room. She knew from all the times that she had taken Katie to the hospital that the side room was where they took you to give you the talk that you didn't necessarily want to hear. Like before, she only perceived a few words coming from the nurse's mouth. "Trying to determine injuries...bleeding out of control... losing blood...going into emergency surgery."

Virginia's parents had arrived and they, along with Virginia and Katie were led to the trauma unit. Suddenly, a group of nurses came running down the hall. One of them began pushing the elevator button with panic.

"Stand back!" A nurse held out her arms and pushed Virginia and her family out of the hallway and into the waiting room behind them. Virginia looked down the hall and saw a swarm of doctors running next to a patient being rolled down the hallway. The patient was covered with a bloody sheet and had a severely swollen, bruised face covered in blood. Still, Virginia recognized Aaron in a split second.

"That's my husband!" She screamed. The nurse, still holding Virginia back with her arms, froze. Virginia's eyes got as big as saucers.

Dr. Kensor, a trauma surgeon at Vanderbilt, came over to Virginia and held her arms and looked her in the eyes. "I'm not going to lie, it doesn't look good," he said squeezing her arms. "We have to get the bleeding to stop, it's really crucial." He turned and looked back at Aaron. "I'm sorry but I have to go." He sped off to attend to her husband.

I was on call at Vanderbilt that afternoon and at the time I received notice of Aaron's arrival, I was told that he probably wasn't going to make it. I rushed over to the hospital. As I changed into scrubs and examined Aaron, I reflected on the overwhelming threat to his life – his injuries almost made survival seem insurmountable. Aaron had multiple fractures - his legs, pelvis, arms, and the base of his spine. He was also undergoing hemorrhagic shock from extensive bleeding in his left thigh.

But as I went to speak with Virginia, I thought about my own family. Watching Virginia hold Katie in her arms I imagined a life without my father in Hillsboro and how much Katie would miss as she grew up. The love and support of a father helped shape me, and I wanted the same for this little girl. As Virginia cried I assured her I would do everything in my power to help save her husband. I asked Virginia to have faith and to hold on. I believe that meeting Aaron's daughter was meant to happen – it was a message to me from Above.

Together, Dr. Kensor and I began to control the bleeding by treating the injuries to his veins. As soon as the bleeding was under control, I immediately began to clean his wounds in his pelvis and began stabilizing the bones in his legs.

When you put a patient under anesthesia, you assume that they are unconscious and unaware of what is happening. In cases like Aaron's they often don't even know they had been in an accident. Little did I realize that Aaron was very much aware of the situation.

Aaron later recalled that he heard cheering as if he were in a loud arena. A lady with a British accent began narrating the procedures we were performing, as if she were announcing plays in a game. He felt a warm blanket on his face. Slowly, Aaron began floating up out of his body. As he did so, he looked down and saw himself lying naked on the operating table. His brothers appeared beside him.

"Dude!" said Lucas, "Check that out. Oh my God!"

By 2 a.m. the surgery was over. Aaron was in critical condition. It was very likely that he wouldn't make it through the night. We decided to take him off all medications to determine if he had any brain activity. My surgical team and I all stood around Aaron's bed, along with Virginia, hoping and praying that he would wake up.

Aaron was barely recognizable to Virginia. His face was swollen, and he was wrapped in bandages like a mummy. Virginia sat next to her husband, pushed back his hair, and whispered in his ear. Aaron slightly nodded his head. Virginia began crying. We knew at that moment he would make it through the night.

When I got home early that morning, I watched Maya sleeping and thanked God for all that I have and for the fact that Aaron made it through surgery. I thought about the long road ahead for his family and what it would take to get Aaron back on his feet.

In the next couple days Aaron had more emergency trauma surgeries. His jaw was wired shut, and he had plates put in both wrists. My colleagues and I stabilized nearly every bone in his arms and legs with plates and rods.

Aaron fell in and out of consciousness during this time. When he'd wake, he'd always see Virginia sitting at his side. In those moments, he knew he needed help beyond what the doctors could give him; he needed prayer. He thought of his co-worker Alec, who said the most beautiful prayers for him. Aaron still couldn't talk.

Virginia sat at Aaron's side, caressing his hand. He slowly lifted his fingers and laid them on her palms. He began to write out Alec's name with his finger. Virginia looked at him, confused.

"God?" she replied.

He tried again. A…L…E…C.

"Job? Are you worried about your job?" She asked.

Aaron furrowed his brow with frustration. That made Virginia smile. His annoyance was a sign that it was still her Aaron behind all those bandages. While he couldn't explain it, Aaron could feel Alec's prayers for him and the family.

Aaron wanted more than anything to see his daughter Katie, but she wasn't allowed in the trauma unit. Virginia would hold up her phone to show Katie her father. She was careful to not show any of his injuries below his face. Seeing her father in that condition would have terrified Katie.

Every time he came out of surgery, Aaron experienced terrible hallucinations. Some days, he imagined he was being whisked off by helicopters to the jungles. Other days, he thought he was literally in hell. He would forget everything that had happened on that fateful day, and Virginia would have to remind him. There was only one thing Aaron wanted to know every time. "Was it my fault?"

"No, honey, you did everything right," Virginia would whisper.

About a week after the accident, I began yet another surgery on Aaron's left leg. It required cleaning of his open wound and a skin graft.

As he lay on the operating table, Aaron's spirit was dark and he was scared. He felt like he was drowning and knew that he was near death. He had his Bible with him; it was black and in bold gold letters the name Jesus was written on the front cover. Somehow, Aaron was able to fling it across the room where it remained on the floor, up against the wall. He fixed his eyes to it, knowing that he was looking at the word of God. Loudly, he began to praise Jesus, just like he did that time he was filled with the Holy Spirit. At that moment, he knew that Jesus would get him out of surgery alive.

During the next several surgeries, Aaron had the same experience. Each time, he had his black Bible with him and he prayed to Jesus as loud as he could. The last time this happened, Aaron was scared. He was hurting and he felt like he was drowning, gasping for air with every breath. He was terrified. He continued to praise Jesus. "Thank you Jesus, thank you for everything you have given me."

Aaron knew he was dying. He was lifted out of his body and floated out of the operating room, through the ceiling, and into the night sky. He flew over Tennessee, and continued floating for what felt like hours. Finally, he stopped at a cliff side overlooking the expansive ocean. There was a great white mist rising from the ocean which enveloped him. Aaron felt its warm embrace and knew in a second that it was God.

"Thank you God," he yelled boldly. "Thank you Lord for

everything you've given me and taking me into your embrace." Aaron felt bathed in peace. He knew death was near, but he wasn't scared.

"If this is my time Lord, I am ready," he assured God. "But Lord, if there's more for me to do on Earth, please let me stay."

Aaron opened his eyes. Virginia was sitting in the chair beside him, holding his hand and resting her head on his bed as she slept. He was back in the hospital. God had returned him to Earth.

From that moment on, Aaron had no hallucinations. Around the hospital, he began to be known as the "Miracle Man." With each surgery came greater risk that Aaron would not wake up or that he would contract a deadly infection, but Aaron knew God was watching over him. He would heal him so that Aaron could finish his work on Earth.

When Christians around the world heard of the "miracle man," they began to say prayers for Aaron. "We got one from Canada today! Another one from England – oh, Katie's friend's sister in Africa is praying for us today!" Virginia squealed with delight as she added countries to her running tally.

Aaron was finally able to see Katie when he moved out of the trauma intensive care unit and onto a normal hospital floor after a few weeks. Katie's face lit up when she saw her father, and the two of them began to cry with happiness. She sat next to him the rest of the day, feeding him ice chips with a spoon.

Aaron was moved to Select Specialty Hospital for rehabilitation. He would be cared for by the nurses there and would return to Vanderbilt only when he needed additional surgeries. From the moment they arrived there, Virginia took over his care. She would clean and re-dress his wounds, change his beddings, bathe him, and wash his hair. The nurses would insist that they should be the ones taking care of Aaron, but she remained firm. When they took their vows in Alaska, she had promised to love him through sickness and in health. She would never let go of that promise.

Virginia's dedication to Aaron was one of the most powerful assets in his road to recovery. Having seen many patients with near life ending trauma, I had come to see the powerful role of family support in helping patients recover. In fact, I had seen it in my own family. As my father was in and out of hospitals when I was a kid it was my mother who not only maintained a busy career delivering babies, but was by my dad's side at every minute and until the end. Without her, my father wouldn't have survived as long as he did.

Virginia was the perfect care-giver. She never left Aaron's side for more than a moment. He was still unable to eat solid foods, so Virginia was given a blender she used to liquefy everything. A nutritionist would come in every few days and monitor Aaron's meals. When she noticed several copies of a book called By Jesus's 39 Stripes, We Were Healed, containing scriptures and prayers beside Aaron's bed she gave a knowing smile. She pointed to the book. "That's why you guys are doing so well, and that's what's making the difference," she said.

"Can I take a few of these books?" She asked. "I have a couple of patients that I'd like to pass these on to."

As Aaron's story spread across the state, reporters from Tennessee came to the hospital to write stories on the "Miracle Man." The other patients watched as photographers flashed their cameras as Aaron worked out on one of the therapy machines, wondering who this man with long hair was and why everybody was talking about him.

Aaron stayed at Select Specialty for two months. By the time he was discharged, he had undergone several additional surgeries. Due to a laceration near his colon, he required a colostomy. His stool was collected in a bag that would have to be emptied and cleaned by Virginia every day.

Preparing their modest home for Aaron's arrival was a major task. He was still in a wheelchair, so Virginia's stepfather had built a ramp to their door. They moved their couch to the motorcycle trailer, which was now empty, and it was replaced by a hospital bed. Virginia got to the house mere minutes before the ambulance arrived with her husband. With her stepfather they were making last minute adjustments just as he arrived. Aaron's bed was situated in the center of the living room and the recliner was placed directly beside it.

For the next few months, Virginia literally lived in that recliner next to her husband. She would bathe him in the kitchen and change his colostomy bag every day. She used a slide board to move him from his hospital bed to his wheelchair. She traded vehicles with her mom, so she would have a large van to transport him.

Life had completely changed for Aaron and Virginia. Katie had moved in with her grandparents while Aaron was at the hospital and rehab, but when Aaron returned home, Katie moved back in as well. Their family was once again together. Several times during his recovery, Aaron had to be rushed to Vanderbilt for emergency surgery. He had poor circulation and a lot of swelling in his legs that would pain him every day, and as the pain continued, Aaron began to become overcome with darkness once again.

With Aaron bed-ridden and with Virginia now his full-time nurse neither had been able to work since the accident, and medical bills from both hospitals began to pile up on the kitchen table. Because Aaron was returning from a work-related task on the day of his accident, worker's compensation kicked in and started paying him two-thirds of his salary for the year. Still, the income was not enough to pay the exorbitant bills that were arriving at their house in large piles each day.

Virginia sat at the kitchen table, tears streaming down her face as she held up a stack of bills, "What are we going to do?" She cried desperately.

At that very moment, the phone rang. It was Aaron's boss, Bobby.

"Hi Aaron," he began when Virginia passed the phone to her husband. "Look, I've been thinking about this a lot, and I've prayed about it several times. I am going to pay everything that worker's compensation doesn't cover. It is the right thing to do."

Aaron began to tear up. When he told Virginia, she began to cry with happiness.

Aaron knew that it was God who once again was saving him and his family.

"Virginia," he said, "It's time to go to church."

Many of my patients were faced with the same struggle that Aaron and Virginia were dealing with – the costs of long hospital stays and multiple surgeries adding up with no end in sight. I never understood why trauma always targeted those just trying to get by and make an honest living, sometimes living paycheck to paycheck. But time after time it was the community that came through to help and lend a helping hand in times of need. The power of community that I first witnessed on a baseball field as a boy was the same force that was making a difference in Aaron's life and so many of my patients.

Virginia began her routine of getting Aaron ready to travel in the van. She would slide him from the hospital bed into the wheelchair with the sliding board. She would place a ramp outside of the van's open doors and carefully wheel him up the ramp and into the car seat. Once Aaron was comfortable, she would break down the ramp and stow it in the back of the van. She would then reverse the process to get him out of the van.

When Virginia rolled Aaron through the doors of the church, everyone stood and began clapping, giving him a standing ovation. Aaron began to tear up. Virginia rolled him over to the edge of the aisle, and the service began.

As Aaron sat and watched the preacher deliver his service, he began to feel somber. He desperately wanted to be back on the stage with his church brothers and sisters, performing music for his church. Virginia looked over at Aaron and just by glancing at his face she knew what he was thinking. She squeezed his hand.

A few weeks later, Aaron got a call from his brother, Lucas. "I've seen how much this has been a struggle for you Aaron. Ethan and I want to throw a benefit for you downtown. And the EMTs who were there at your accident want to organize a motorcycle run benefit." Aaron was delighted. He now had a date in mind for when he would get back on stage and start playing his bass – the day of the benefit, July 14. His arms had been in casts for a long time, which made it hard for him to even pick up his bass. Still, Aaron spent the next few weeks in his bed practicing.

By the time July 14 rolled around, Aaron was ready. With the support of his brothers, Aaron was pulled up on stage in his wheelchair and he began to play. Virginia stood off to the side with David, the music director at their church. They looked at Aaron, then at each other, and both began to cry.

"I think he's ready to start playing at church," said Virginia.

"I think he is too," agreed David.

Throughout this time, Aaron continued to visit me at the clinic. At first, every six weeks and then once he got better, every three months. When I would check Aaron's injuries, I was shocked by the great progress he was making.

"From my perspective, it is amazing how far you've come," I told him. Right from the moment of his accident, everything had fallen in place to ensure that Aaron Matthews would live. From the officer who began praying, the fact that experienced EMTs Joseph and Andrew were both there at the scene of the accident, even the fact that the Vanderbilt Life Flight helicopter was unable to reach him due to an impending storm. Ironically, Life Flight wouldn't have had enough blood onboard to keep him alive, so without that stop at Sumner Regional Medical Center, Aaron would have bled out and died before getting to Vanderbilt. It didn't take any of us very long to know that someone was watching over Aaron that day.

Through the roughest seas, Aaron was anchored by his faith and in the darkest moments his family and community stood by his side. I shared a powerful connection with Aaron and his family as these same forces played such a strong role in shaping my own life – in fact, without faith, family, and the people of Hillsboro I would never have been in a position to help Aaron.

A few weeks after Aaron's benefit, Highland Park Church was holding its regular Sunday morning service and people were milling around as usual prior to the service saying hello to their friends when someone looked up and saw Aaron with his bass in hand and yelled, "Aaron's Back!" Crying, clapping, and cheers erupted.

The entire church fell silent, waiting to hear what would happen next.

Their pastor began his sermon with pictures of Aaron's accident. He showed the x-rays and pictures of him recovering after the surgery. Everyone gasped at the gruesome pictures. He talked about the miracle that everybody already knew had occurred. There was thunderous applause after he finished.

"And now, live on the stage – Aaron Matthews and the church band!"

One year after Aaron's accident, on a warm summer day Maya and I walked through the doors of Highland Park Church. It was their annual Coffee House, an informal event where folks bring food and listen to bands with members from the church performing. There was a lot of buzz and excitement going on when I went in. I saw Aaron standing at the stage with his brothers, setting up their instruments. When he looked over and saw us, he smiled widely and began to wave.

Virginia had invited us to come and surprise Aaron at his one-year anniversary performance. Aaron had improved quickly and he was walking. He still had a few surgeries left to go, but I knew he would get through them just fine.

The lights began to dim, and we all sat down and looked up at Aaron and his band. We began clapping.

"Thank you all for coming," Aaron began as the applause died down. "As you know, it has been one year exactly since my accident. The day after it happened, I was supposed to be up on this stage, playing with my brothers. I'm sorry for being late," he joked. "I got a little caught up, but I'm here now."

Everyone laughed. "I had some dark moments lying in the hospital bed at Vanderbilt. I would cry out to God and ask why. Why do I have to go through this? When I see you all here today, I think I am getting a sense of God's plan, and why he kept me here."

He paused and looked around the room at his church. Aaron had a connection to each and every person there. Not one of them would have been impacted in the same way if this accident had happened to anyone else. He had that special link to each and all.

Aaron continued. "I've had a lot of people tell me what an inspiration I've been to them, just helping them get through troubling days, thinking, 'at least I'm not Aaron Matthews.'"

Everyone laughed again.

"And today, I want to thank you all for the unconditional love and support that you've given me. I especially want to thank my doctor, Dr. Sethi. When they told him on that fateful day that I was going to die before morning, he knew they were wrong. God had other plans for me." He strummed his bass.

As Aaron spoke I looked at my wife who was pregnant with our boy and tears started to flow down my face as I realized the incredible privilege of being a doctor. Aaron had come so far and I had been a part of it. I thought about my dad and how proud he would have been to see this moment– a life that I had helped save. But it was Aaron's faith in God, the love of Virginia and Katie, and his community that did the heavy lifting. Moments like these made me realize how as Tennesseans our lives are all connected regardless of the differences in our life stories. Without the sacrifices my parents had made to leave their country for my brother and me, Aaron and I would probably never have met.

"This song is dedicated to all of you." Aaron began to strum his guitar and play. And we all looked up at Aaron and basked in the Supreme Love and Graciousness that allowed that special moment to happen.

Progress Notes on Aaron

Aaron now works as the parts manager for a service and interior shop doing what he loves. His pastor built him a desk that gives Aaron the ability to sit or stand at his desk, allowing him to work painlessly throughout the day. He continues to play bass at his church every Sunday and around Nashville every month. Aaron and Virginia have begun volunteering at the Trauma Survivors Network at Vanderbilt, where he inspires trauma patients with his own story of survival and recovery.

Michael

The tiny bell over the door echoed loudly as Michael walked into the tobacco outlet. He walked down the familiar path through the aisles to the refrigerators in the back. He opened the door and pulled out his favorite brand of beer, to which he had developed an almost religious loyalty. He casually walked up to the counter to pay for his beer and pick up a pack of cigarettes, but when his gaze shifted to the new store clerk, he froze. Her short, blonde hair delicately framed her face, and her warm smile gave him butterflies in his stomach. The name tag said her name was Madison.

"Hi Madison," Michael said with a bright smile.

"Hello," she responded politely. He saw her look down at the gold band on his left ring finger as she scanned his six-pack.

Michael felt that perhaps she had misjudged him and he wished he could spill out his entire story to her at that moment. He would tell her that although he was legally married, they had long since separated. That no matter how many times he asked for a divorce, she refused to part amicably and allow each to move on with their lives. Michael considered himself a good, but lost Christian.

Michael and his wife Nicole's biggest problem in their marriage were their different views regarding faith and religion. He always felt that if he went to church, he could get the support he needed to break an addiction to drugs that both of them had struggled with but unlike Nicole, Michael wanted to be saved – and to be sober. Although his parents weren't religious, Michael's grandparents would drag the family to church quite often while he was growing up. As a young boy, Michael didn't see the power in religion or faith that could change his life. When his family moved to Nashville when he was a teenager, he fell in with the wrong crowd in high school and it was then that he began experimenting with drugs and began going down a treacherous path. It was also when he met Nicole. At the young age of eighteen, Nicole and Michael married right out of high school. He started his own painting company. But with every year that passed, he began to feel as if he were drowning in sin. Nicole embodied the destructive lifestyle that Michael was desperately trying to avoid.

He tried to convince her that the two of them should start going to church on Sundays, but she refused. Michael felt trapped in their marriage and hopeless about his future.

And then there was Madison. Over the next few weeks, Michael began going to the tobacco outlet not for the cigarettes, but to talk to Madison. Over time, he explained his situation to her during their brief encounters at the store. He talked to Madison about his internal wrestling with his faith. He was happy to learn that she too was interested in being Saved by God. He dreamt of how nice it would be to raise a devout, Christian family that went to church together on Sundays while working hard to achieve their dreams. Michael remained in a deep pit of darkness and depression.

After three years of seeing Michael in the outlet every week, Madison became concerned when he stopped coming to the store. She prayed that he had been able to overcome his sinful addiction, but also worried that something terrible might have happened. The two of them had grown to become close friends, and she wondered why he would disappear without saying a word. After months of not seeing him, she was shocked when he came back into the store, without a ring on his finger.

"Hi Madison," Michael said warmly. "With God's good grace, I've been given the chance to turn my life around. Nicole and I divorced a few months ago, and I've been working to change my old, bad habits. I never want to step foot in this store again, except to see you."

Madison smiled shyly.

"Would you like to go out for dinner tonight?" he asked.

She smiled. "I get off at eight."

That night, Michael took Madison out to a local diner. They had burgers and shared a large milkshake. Although they hadn't seen each other in months, they both felt that the other had never left their life. Since that night, Michael and Madison never spent another day apart.

Michael fell totally in love with Madison. Within the year, they were married, and Madison became pregnant with their first child. For the next decade of Michael's life, he lived the devout Christian life of which he had always dreamed. He began taking his family to Granville Methodist, where his parents attended church. Following the Lord's message, he began volunteering in his community. He volunteered as a tour guide for a southern store called The Garage, where he would share the history of cars that was deeply embedded in the history of Granville, a small town about sixty-five miles east of Nashville. As his son, Paul, grew older, he began to follow his parents everywhere, like a shadow.

"When we see one of you, we know the other two can't be far behind," his friends would joke when Michael's family headed out for the lake to their boat. They would all go fishing together and eventually, Madison began working with Michael at his company. The painting business he had created more than a decade ago had transformed into a garage door company. Madison originally had planned to help out for only a day or two a week while they looked for an additional man to hire, but Michael quickly learned that Madison was a better employee than any man who ever worked with him. Madison and Michael were practically inseparable. They were more than just best friends – they were soul mates.

And then one day, it was as if the switch for the light that had shone brightly on his life had been turned off. As the economy spiraled into a recession, the phones at their business stopped ringing. Michael decided he needed to get another job and began to look for work across Tennessee, but his prospects were dismal. He soon realized that he might have to move his family out of his beloved state where he had spent his entire life. Two months after he finished his last job with his garage company, Michael and his family moved to West Virginia. He found work at a phone line company for a few years, but he always had the feeling that the job wasn't stable. He began to see a potential and disastrous trend in his future of moving from job to job, traveling around the country and never truly having a permanent home. Not only did the stress of trying to support his family with such an unstable lifestyle scare him, but he realized how hard it would be to establish himself at a church and feared succumbing to his old, bad habits.

After two years with the phone line company, Michael lost his job. Luckily, his parents had just opened a marina back in Granville and needed extra help running their new business. They invited Michael and his family to come live with them, and they could all work together to build the business. Michael moved back to Tennessee, hopeful for the future. But during their first season, the marina barely made enough money to stay afloat.

"Looks like we'll have to go into the good old construction business, son," his father said the day they locked up the doors to their marina for the last time.

Michael became overcome with worry, and began slipping back into his old habits. After Madison and Paul would fall asleep each night, Michael would quietly go down to the kitchen, open a few beers and drink his sorrows away. By the end of the summer, the construction work fizzled out, and Michael was once again looking for work.

"What if we started working for a housing development company?" His younger brother Ryan asked. "They always seem to be looking for help."

"I don't know Ryan," Michael said reluctantly. "That seems like a risky job."

"Why do you think they're always looking for workers? Nobody wants to do it, but somebody has to."

Michael sighed. He was desperate. "Okay," he agreed finally.

Sure enough, it didn't take long for Ryan and Michael to find a company to work for and they began working on building a new house. Over the next few months, Ryan and Michael worked together every day. Although they were no longer children, Michael still felt protective over his younger brother. Whenever there was a potentially risky job, Michael always offered to do it. When they got to the roofing part of the construction though, both were wary about working so high off the ground. One day, Michael suggested to John, his supervisor, a safer way of moving from one side of the roof to the other.

"That's not the way we do it," John responded.

"I'm sorry, but I don't feel comfortable with the way we currently do it. I don't think it's safe." Michael said.

"Either do it the way I do it, or don't do it at all," John said angrily.

Michael sighed and made his way up to the roof. As he precariously crouched on the slanted rooftop, he began to place shingles, one by one in a neat square. Once he was done with one side, he stood up and made his way over to the other side. He raised his leg to step over a set of shingles.

As he stepped, the toe board under his foot that was supporting him gave way, and Michael lost his balance and with visions of Madison and Paul flashing before him, began toppling over the edge.

Michael desperately and unsuccessfully tried to grab onto anything and everything he could. As he fell off the side of the roof, he managed to roll to his side and hit the ground with a sickening thud. When he hit, he rolled uncontrollably and violently into the tires of an eighteen-foot supply trailer that was parked next to the house. His leg slammed into the tire, making a large cracking sound. He lay frozen on the ground.

Ryan ran around the trailer to his older brother with a look of terror on his face. He looked down at Michael's leg and his face drained of all color. "I'm going to call 911," he sputtered.

"I'll do it," said John, who had also run over, his hands shaking.

"Do you want me to call Madison?" Ryan asked.

"No, no, no, don't call her," said Michael quickly, lifting his head up off the ground. "I'll go to the hospital and the doctors will probably just cast me up tonight. Then I'll go home and explain to her what happened," Michael said, trying but failing to sound hopeful.

"Michael," began Ryan, shaking his head. "I don't think you're going home tonight."

Michael laid his head back down on the ground, breathing heavily.

"Your leg doesn't even look like a leg!" Ryan said.

Michael looked at his leg and reached down to touch it.

"No, don't do that!" Ryan warned.

"Why? Is there anything sticking out?"

"No. But it just looks funny. Don't worry though, everything will be fine," said Ryan. His voice betrayed his own fear.

"Go to the truck and get some water and rags. Maybe wipe off some of the blood." Michael said, starting to feel light-headed. Ryan hurried off toward the truck.

The next few minutes while they waited for the paramedics to arrive felt like hours. When Michael finally heard the sirens, he breathed a sigh of relief. Three paramedics jumped out of the ambulance and rushed toward him.

"If one of you will give me your arm I'll try to pick myself up," he told them.

Two of paramedics reached down and grabbed Michael's hand, lifting him up. He led out a blood-curdling scream. The pain in his leg was unbearable. He continued screaming as they put him into the ambulance and closed the door. Michael was beginning to lose consciousness from the pain. For the next half hour, he remained in this halfway state, aware of the pain in his leg but unable to register what was happening around him. When the ambulance doors finally opened at the Cookeville Regional Medical Center, he saw his dad and Madison standing there. Her face was covered in tears.

"Madison," Michael murmured. "Where's Paul?"

"He's with your mom," she said tearfully. The paramedics began wheeling Michael in to the emergency room. Michael closed his eyes, his mind and body both numbed with pain. He heard voices talking around him, but he couldn't open his eyes to see what was going on. He finally lifted his eyelids ever so slightly and looked up at the sky. He was still outside, not in the hospital. He saw a man in a white coat standing next to his stretcher, talking to Madison and Ryan.

There's nothing I can do for him here, I'm really sorry," Michael heard the doctor say.

Over Michael's loud sobs, he heard the doctor say the word "Vanderbilt Hospital."

"Vanderbilt," Madison said, nodding her head. "We want to go there."

"It'll be a long ride," the doctor warned. He looked down at Michael. "Hang in there; you're going to be okay."

They lifted the stretcher into the ambulance, slammed the doors and headed off to Nashville, with the sirens blaring. The next hour was the longest hour of Michael's life. He continued to drift in and out of consciousness. Still, he could feel someone squeezing his hand tightly the whole time, and he knew Madison was at his side.

I had received a call from the doctor in Cookeville that a trauma patient was headed our way and by the time Michael had entered the ER, I was there to meet him. When I saw him come in through those doors, I knew he was in for a long ride.

"I'm Dr. Sethi," I said to Madison. "I'll be taking care of your husband. Everything will be fine." She nodded while Michael looked up at me hazily. "I'm going to take him into the operating room and I will come out and give you an update immediately afterward," I continued. "Thank you Dr. Sethi," Madison whispered. "Please take good care of him."

The paramedics wheeled Michael to the radiograph machine so we could get x-rays of his leg before we prepped him for surgery. When I saw his x-rays, I understood the severity of his injuries and the threat to his leg. He had multiple fractures and his knee was broken into many small pieces. He was developing compartment syndrome which effectively cut off the blood flow to his leg. We immediately took him to the operating room to try and save his leg.

As I scrubbed my hands at the sink I felt my nerves. I was two years into practice and this was potentially one of the worst injuries I had ever seen. I desperately wanted to save Michael's leg and to help his family. Strangely during times like this I found my mind wondering back to that cold foggy night when my parents left India and everything they knew behind for an unknown future and for their unborn children. That level of sacrifice demonstrated real audacity and bravery and it was that kind of courage that I needed now. We operated that night for six hours and saved Michael's leg, at least for the meanwhile.

When Michael woke the next morning, he looked around his hospital room with confusion. When he saw the external fixator on his leg, which was swollen to double the size, his eyes became wide. "Madison," he murmured. "Where's Madison?"

"I'm right here," said Madison, who was standing near the window. She rushed toward Michael; her eyes welled up with tears. She held his hand.

"What happened," he asked softly.

Madison began telling Michael the entire story. He slowly began to regain his memories of the accident. A few minutes later, I entered his room and began explaining to Michael what had happened to his leg. I told him that he had a severe fracture to his knee and bad injuries to his foot and ankle. While it was hard to tell him, I explained that he was at high risk for an above knee amputation and that we would have to work closely together to save his leg. As the tears flowed from Michael's eyes I told him to have faith and to imagine one year from now when this was all over, no matter what the outcome, he needed to be able to look back and say he had given it all he had to save his leg.

Over the next few days my partners and I performed multiple procedures on him in the operating room, all of which were successful.

Michael felt hopeless. He wondered if, after all these surgeries, his leg would still end up being amputated. He hated seeing both Madison and Paul going through this. Paul was still too young to visit his father in the trauma unit, and Michael was sure the young boy was terrified waiting at home worrying what was happening to his father.

"Dr. Sethi, you should just cut it off and be done with it," he said with exasperation a few days later. I was in his room talking with him and Madison about what we would be doing in his next surgery.

I looked him square in the eyes. "Michael, we are not going to do that. If I can save it, I'm going to save it." I could tell that Michael was a fighter – he would do anything to make ends meet for his family and his story was similar to so many families I grew up with in Hillsboro. During tough economic times many folks on the farm would switch to construction to make ends meet and end up getting severely injured in the process. Many times it was my dad who would initially take care of them in the emergency room. Like Michael, all they were only trying to do was to make an honest living so they could support their family. I desperately wanted to help him.

Madison gave a nod of approval. "We have to keep trying, God will watch over you," she said softly.

I gave Michael permission to leave the hospital a few days later. He had a major surgery ahead of him in our effort to save his leg and I wanted him to go home and rest up.

Paul welcomed his father home with open arms and Michael was delighted to be home again. During the next two weeks, Madison focused on helping him in any way she could. In the mornings, she would brush his teeth and give him a sponge bath. She would dress him, make him breakfast, and help him get back into bed to rest. For the entire day, Madison never left his side.

"Let me help, mommy," Paul would say. Although he was only nine, Paul wanted to help Madison with everything.

"You can help dress daddy's leg," she said.

With his wife and son helping, Michael felt he could get through anything. Still, there was something that bothered him. Even though he had always felt the Lord's presence around him, Michael had still never been Saved. Although he could barely move, he wanted more than anything to go back to church and accept the Lord as his savior. He could only hope that one day he would be able to walk into church on his own two feet and have the Lord welcome him with open arms.

Two weeks later, Michael was re-admitted to the hospital for the removal of his external fixator and to fix the fracture in his knee. Over six hours we pieced his leg back together and surgery went well. Despite the surgical success, and due to the gravity of his injury, I was still concerned about the risks of infection.

When Michael woke in his room a few hours after surgery I talked with him about what we had done and told him about the next steps in his recovery.

Michael was ecstatic. He was anxious to be able to walk again. "I wish I had something productive to do during this time," he said when he returned home from the hospital. "I feel so useless just lying here all day."

"Why don't you read the Bible, cover to cover? You always said you wanted to," Madison suggested.

"I know, but to be honest, I don't think I could understand it all," Michael admitted. Madison was silent. She nodded her head and didn't say anything more. A few days later, she handed Michael a book.

"It's an adapted version of the Bible written to make it easier to understand the Word of God."

Indeed, Madison was right. Over the next few days, Michael was absorbed in reading the teachings of the Bible. He wondered what his life would have been like if he had read this Bible earlier in his life, when he was having struggles with his first marriage and his job. Instead of going to his six-pack of beer, he could have opened up the Bible and found the verse that would have instructed him on what to do next. As he read this Bible, Michael felt like he was turning into a totally new person. Although he loved Madison, he never felt comfortable enough to confide his problems with her. His accident made him realize how fragile he really was, and how dependent he was both on his wife and on God. Now, he shared everything.

"I'm worried about the bills that are piling up, with the both of us out of work," he would tell her repeatedly over the next few months.

"I am too," she would admit. "Let's pray."

Michael felt his life was finally coming back together. As the months passed, and as his health continued to improve every time he came to my clinic, I was hopeful, and so was he. When he came down with a fever early in the fall, he became worried.

"We'll put you on antibiotics," I said when he came into clinic after examining the redness around his knee. I was starting to get concerned, but I knew there was nothing we could do but wait.

A week passed, and Michael's fever got worse. "I'm taking you to the emergency room," Madison said, her voice trembling. His leg looked infected, so we admitted Michael and prepared for surgery. As we went to the operating room I was worried for Michael. I realized what this meant to his family. It was also hard for me to take as I had seen so many families in my practice who had lost this fight, and I wanted Michael to win. I thought about Paul and what it would mean for him if his father lost this battle.

When Michael woke, I was standing at the foot of his bed. I explained to him the long surgery he had undergone. I told him I was very optimistic about saving his leg and clearing his infection and that he would be on antibiotics for a long time, maybe even a year. "Thank you Dr. Sethi," he said. "You know, I never made it through the twelfth grade, but hearing you explain everything so simply makes me know that I'm in good hands."

Over the next week we took him to the operating room multiple times to clean his leg. We used a plastic surgeon to move tissue around in order to cover part of the skin that we had removed.

On the day that Michael was going to be discharged from the hospital, he couldn't help but feel depressed. He was still on antibiotics and there was still a chance he would need another reconstructive procedure to cover the wounds. He wondered if he would ever fully recover and be able to go back to work. His relationship with his parents and brother was becoming strained. Not only that, but Madison was taking care of him every moment of the day. He wanted to go back to taking care of her. As he was thinking about all this, Madison walked into the room, snacks in her hand from the hospital cafeteria. When she saw he was awake, she walked over to the bed.

"Do you know what day it is?"

Michael paused for a moment. "No, it's been so hard to keep track of the days in here."

"It's October 13," she said. "Our anniversary."

Tears formed in Michael's eyes. "I'm so sorry Madison, I'm so sorry for forgetting."

"It's okay," she assured him.

"No it's not," he said, his voice trembling. "This is all my fault. The day of the accident, I saw that Ryan was terrified of going up there on the roof; he's scared of heights, so I thought to myself 'I'll do it.' 'He has two kids and I have one, so if something happened to him they would both starve.' And I knew that you would take care of me like no other wife would. I've just been so blessed to have you."

Madison smiled. "And I feel blessed to have you."

"I used to take so many things for granted in my life," Michael continued. "Simple things like hopping out of bed, jumping in the shower and heading off to work. People dread going to work and right now I would love to be able to do that and to be able to go out into the yard and play baseball with Paul."

Madison squeezed Michael's hand. "God does everything for a reason. This accident has brought us closer together and closer to God. It was a terrible thing to happen, but it brought so much good to our life."

"You're right," Michael added. "I don't see life the way I used to. This accident has woken me up."

The day after Michael came home, Madison carefully changed his bandages over his wounds.

"I want to help," Paul said, peering over her shoulder.

"Okay, but you might not like seeing this, Madison warned.

"I don't mind," said Paul, shrugging.

Madison carefully peeled back the bandages, exposing the fresh skin grafts underneath. Michael immediately felt squeamish looking down at his legs. "You don't have to do this," he said quickly. "We should ask to have a nurse."

"Oh stop," said Madison. "I'm fine." She began taking out the gauze that was inserted into the open wounds in his leg, exposing the hardware inside. She cleaned out each wound then repacked it. Paul watched his mother intently, studying her every move. After 10 minutes, the whole ordeal was over, and his leg was covered in clean bandages.

"I can do it tomorrow, mom," Paul said. "After I help dad take a bath."

Michael looked at his son in amazement. When he looked into his eyes, he felt like he was looking at a teenager instead of a child. When did he grow up so quickly?

Over the next few weeks, Michael remained bed-ridden. His leg was getting sorer and sorer, so much so that he could barely move it. When Madison would remove his bandages to clean his wounds, he noticed that he had one open sore that just wasn't healing. He knew that it would take time, and remained hopeful that everything would be okay. That is, until, Madison lifted his covers one day and screamed in terror.

"What's wrong?" Michael said with panic.

"It looks like someone just shot your leg – there's blood everywhere!"

Michael looked down at his leg. Blood was soaking the sheets. Madison ran out of the room, crying, calling for Michael's parents to come upstairs and to call 911. Michael's dad took one look at his leg and turned pale.

The ambulance arrived in minutes. The paramedics ran up the stairs and surveyed Michael's leg. "We checked your chart and it says you have a doctor's appointment on Monday. We can dress your wound now and you can wait until then, or we can take you now."

"Take him now," said Madison and Michael's dad in unison.

Michael was carried down to the ambulance and began the long ride over to Vanderbilt Hospital. There, Dr. Peterson, one of my partners and a plastic surgeon immediately began operating on Michael's leg. The skin flap that had been placed earlier had died and a new skin flap had to be added to cover the large wound.

When Michael woke from surgery, he felt weak. He looked around his room and saw Madison sitting by his side. Her face was tense and she appeared to be in pain. "What's wrong?"

"Now, my leg is hurting," she said while she rubbed it.

"Maybe it's the way you slept?"

"Maybe," she said. "Don't worry about it; I'm sure it'll be fine. Anyway, the plastic surgeon came in earlier and told me that the reconstruction went great. When you're discharged in a few days, a nurse will come by and put an IV into your arm that will deliver antibiotics into your bloodstream so this doesn't happen again."

Michael sighed, "Okay, hopefully this will be my last surgery."

When Michael returned home a few nights later he anxiously awaited the nurse to arrive with his antibiotics. She never came.

"Don't worry, she will be here in the morning," Madison assured him.

That entire night, he couldn't sleep. He imagined that his leg was swarming with bacteria that were slowly eating away at his flesh. He turned to look at Madison, who was also tossing and turning, obviously still in pain from her leg. Michael was terrified of what the future had in store for the two of them. He began to pray. "This is it God," he said. "When I can walk, I'm going back to church. I'm going to be Saved."

The nurse arrived in the morning just as Madison had predicted. As soon as the antibiotics began to course through his veins, Michael breathed a sigh of relief. "I wish there was something we could give you for your leg pain, Madison," he said.

"Don't worry about me," she said. "I need to be here to take care of you."

The pain in Madison's leg was unrelenting. After a week passed the throbbing got worse and Michael knew she had to go to the hospital. "Just go to the doctor honey," he said one morning.

"Fine," she said finally. "I'm sure it's nothing though. Go back to bed."

Michael kissed Madison before she left the house. Then, he closed his eyes and said a prayer, asking God to care for his wife. He drifted off to sleep for the next couple of hours.

When his father returned home without his wife, Michael knew instantly that something was wrong.

"What happened to Madison?"

Michael's dad sat down on the bed next to him. "Now don't worry, but they are going to keep Madison overnight. There was a blood clot in her leg and it moved to her lungs."

Michael lurched up in bed, tears forming in his eyes. "I need to get out of here," he said, grasping at the covers, "I need to go and see her."

Michael's dad pushed him down. "Now hold on a minute, you know that you can't leave with your IV in."

"I don't care!" Michael said, struggling against his father's arms. "I need to go see her, please take me there."

"You know I can't do that, Michael."

Michael stopped pushing and became limp. Then, he reached over to the dresser, grabbed his laptop, and began searching.

"What are you doing?" Michael's father asked.

"I'm looking up what happens when you get a blood clot in your lung."

"Don't do that, you're just going to scare yourself."

Michael knew his father was right. He took a deep breath and began to pray. For the entire day, Michael remained in his bed, praying. Madison was always the one who would tell him that everything would be fine. Now, it was up to him to remind himself that God was watching over them both.

The next couple days without Madison were heart-wrenching. They hadn't spent one day apart since that night in the diner more than a decade ago. Now, they had to be apart at a time when they needed each other the most. In the past, he would have surely reached for a bottle of whisky at a time like this. Now, he looked through the Bible, reading passage after passage. During the next two days, he read the entire Bible. The moment he reached the last page and closed the cover, he heard the door open downstairs. It was Madison. In seconds, she was up the stairs and in Michael's arms. After minutes of holding her close to him, he held back her tears-streaked face and said "Madison, it's time we go back to church."

A few days later, Dr. Peterson gave Michael approval to discontinue his IV antibiotics and the following Sunday he went back to church for the first time since his accident. He was still unable to walk, so Madison pushed him in his wheelchair.

"Let me help," Paul said that morning. His eyes had lit up when his parents told him they were going back to church. When the three of them climbed out of the car and walked up the side ramp to the church doors, Michael's heart beat wildly.

The moment they entered, all eyes turned to face Michael and his family. Church members began to huddle around them, shaking Michael's hand and hugging Madison.

"We're so glad you're back."

"Really, just a blessing."

"A living miracle!"

Michael beamed up at them. "Soon enough, I'll be walking into church on my own two feet. I'll be doing laps around Granville!"

They all laughed. "I can't wait until you do," chimed in Pastor Bill.

When Michael went to his first physical therapy session the next week, he was anxious to get started.

"How soon before I'll be able to walk?" Michael asked his therapist, Beth.

"Well Michael, I'll say it like this – you'll know my grandkids and I'll know yours by the time this is over."

Michael sighed. He wanted more than anything to walk again. He would do anything to be able to go back to work and provide for his family. "I can and I will," said Michael, repeating the motto his father had professed to him all his life. Michael knew that without his family, his doctors, and God, there was no way he would be able to walk again. Having their support made him stronger than he ever thought he could be. He knew there was one more step he had to take before he could take a real step with his own two feet.

"Madison, I want to get baptized," Michael said when he came home from therapy that day. She smiled. "I think it's time. I'll call Pastor Bill."

That Sunday, it seemed like the entire community of Granville was at church. The room was buzzing with excitement, but the crowd quieted down when Pastor Bill approached the podium and announced Michael's baptism. Normally, the baptisms took place at the lake down the road. But because Michael was still at risk of infection, the baptism would take place within the church.

"Would you like to get dripped or poured?" Pastor Bill asked as he stood next to the tub of holy water.

"I don't care," Michael answered, shrugging his shoulders. His eyes were glistening with tears, "As long as it happens."

In the seconds following the first drop of water falling on Michael's forehead, he knew his life had changed forever. On the darkest days it was Michael's faith and Madison's love that sustained him and moved him forward to this point.

Although Madison usually went to therapy with Michael, her friend, Lily, was in town on Michael's birthday so the two of them dropped Michael off at therapy before they went grocery shopping. He figured he had about an hour before they came back.

"You're working really hard today," Beth said toward the end of the session, clearly impressed.

"I'm going to walk today," he told Beth with determination in his voice. When he had become baptized a few weeks earlier, he had asked God to help him take his first steps forward on December 31, the last day of a life-changing year. It was also his birthday.

Beth smiled, "Okay, we've been doing your exercises for an hour now, let's see what you got." She helped Michael stand up using his walker. Although it pained him to bear weight on his feet, he was able to steady himself.

"If you're comfortable doing it, you can let go of your walker now."

Just as he was getting ready to let go, Michael saw that Madison and Lily had returned from the store. Madison had just gotten out of the car and was looking through the large window into the therapy office. She froze when she saw Michael standing, and they locked eyes. In one swift moment, Michael pushed his walker away from him. With his eyes transfixed on Madison, he began to walk forward.

"You did it!" Beth exclaimed. "You're walking!"

The look on Madison's face was priceless. As he got closer to the window, he saw that her face was covered in tears. He smiled at her. "Thank you, Jesus," he whispered.

Over the next month, Michael was determined to walk further and further. Madison had gotten a cane to use after she was hospitalized with the blood clot in her leg and now that she didn't need it, he could use it as he practiced. His next appointment to see me was in February, and he was determined to walk into my office.

Michael was a true believer. He knew that if he wanted it, he could get it with help from God. What surprised him was how easy it was to talk to God. He talked to Him the way he talked to Madison, or anyone else he met. He had never thought he could have a relationship like this with his Savior. Even more, he knew that God was watching over him through his church.

Pastor Bill and a few other members of the church began planning a benefit charity auction. "I know it must be a great struggle to pay the hospital bills for both yours and Madison's conditions, especially with both of you out of work. It's our duty as Christians to help," said Pastor Bill at church that Sunday.

Michael wept with happiness. The next few weeks flew by, and soon it was time for Michael's next appointment in the trauma clinic. I reviewed his chart in my office before walking to his room. Halfway through the hallway, I froze. There was Michael, walking slowly but surely down the hallway toward me.

I usually try to hide emotion but in this second I couldn't hold back the tears – it meant so much to me. Michael had fought so hard to get to this point, and I thanked God for the privilege to share it with him. In that moment I looked at Paul and I thought about what this would mean for him. Would he one day many years from now look upon his father's journey as a lesson in courage and the power of faith and family?

Michael came up and began to walk circles around me. "I can walk doc!" He responded. He stopped and stood in front of me, and gave me a big hug. "Thank you Dr. Sethi, for helping me walk again. You gave me my life back. There is no way I can ever repay you. I will forever be in your debt."

"Now, there is something else that I need to ask you," Michael said. "Madison's aunt surprised us with a trip to Myrtle Beach. I haven't gone on a vacation in thirteen years. I was wondering if it would be possible for me to go?" he asked nervously.

I gave him a pat on his shoulder. "If you think you can do it, I want you to do it."

Michael nodded. "I know I can."

Michael knew he wasn't the same person he was a year earlier, or even 10 years ago when he walked into that tobacco outlet and met Madison for the first time. Every time he went to church, his friends would call him a "walking miracle." He knew he could have died that day when he fell thirty-eight feet off that roof. But he felt that God wasn't done with him, that He had a different plan. He just had to figure out what it was.

As Michael stood at the very edge of the water a week later in Myrtle Beach, he looked out at the deep, vast ocean, and felt a sense of peace overcome him. Madison stood at his side, clutching his hand tightly.

"Did you think we'd be standing here one year ago?" she asked softly.

"No," he said honestly. "But then again, I was lost one year ago. I needed to be Saved, and I was. God could have tapped me on the shoulder, but instead, he pushed me off a roof."

And with that, he and Madison began to walk on the sandy beach, one step at a time.

Progress Notes on Michael

Michael continued to recover with help from his wife, Madison and his son Paul, who has continued to grow fast. He is almost back to normal and will soon be able to go back to work. He and his family recently bought their own house in West Virginia on the street where Madison grew up with her entire family. While she continues to look for work, they are happy to be back in the warm embraces of family and have their support as they move forward with their lives.

Kristen

Kristen sat in her grandmother's lap as she rocked back and forth. She held a card she had received from her father for her 11th birthday. Gazing down at the image of a happy father and daughter on the cover, her grandmother squeezed her tightly.

"Don't worry Kristen, God will take care of us."

For the second time that year, Kristen's father had returned to Colorado, where she was living, demanding to see his daughter. Her mother's rule was he had to be sober when he visited. He never was. Still, he would come determined to take Kristen with him and several times he had tried to kidnap her. Now, whenever her mother knew he would be in town, she sent Kristen to her grandmother's house for safe keeping.

Kristen knew all the stories that her mother and half-brother, Carson, had told her about their father, who was an abusive and raging alcoholic. When her mother was pregnant with Kristen, her father had kicked her so hard the doctors were sure Kristen would be born brain dead or severely damaged. Even after she was born, the abuse continued. When she was three, she remembered her brother stepping in between Kristen's drunken father and their mother and chasing him out of the house with a butcher knife. Despite all the stories and all she had seen, Kristen still wanted to know her father. Now, at the age of 11, she wished more than anything that she could be a part of one happy family and have a father who was sober and loving and always there for her.

She was shocked to learn that less than two months after her father had come looking for her the last time, he had died from pneumonia and the very next day, her grandmother passed away. Kristen was numb with pain. Her mother, who was a strong Christian woman and had learned quickly how to double as both parents, helped her through the next few months. "Grandma is home with God now," she would whisper to Kristen as she kissed her and put her to bed.

Over the next few years, life became much harder for Kristen. She was diagnosed with scoliosis at thirteen, as she entered high school. She had a large rod put into her back and was in a cast for several months. The teasing at school was nearly as bad as the incredible pain from the rod that kept slipping, which created even further problems with her back. To avoid the bullying, she began being home-schooled, and luckily for Kristen, her mother was always there to support her.

"Once you get your rod off, you can do anything you want," her mother would remind her. Sure enough, Kristen's scoliosis improved within the year, and she was back in school in no time. For the rest of high school, Kristen was a star in her class. She was an honors student and began playing sports. Every Sunday morning at 10 without fail, her family went to church. Sitting in her stiff, stuffy dress as the pastor droned on in words that Kristen didn't understand did nothing to ignite her faith, or her brother's for that matter. Her brother Carson experimented with drugs and many times in the middle of the night, Kristen and her mother would receive a phone call from the police station; it would be Carson asking them to bail him out of jail.

"You need to get help," Kristen would plead with her brother.

Carson tried going to rehab for his drug addiction, but every time he finished rehab he found himself surrounded by darkness once again. One day on a sudden whim, he decided to move to Hollywood and try to make it big in the music industry. Kristen wished the best for her brother but feared the worse. As she expected, she heard the soft, familiar slur in his voice every time she talked with him on the phone. Even the phone calls stopped one day. Carson had become homeless and could no longer afford a place to live, let alone a cell phone. Several months after losing touch with her brother, Kristen received an unexpected phone call.

"Come visit me during school break," said Carson, with a tone of excitement. "I have someone I want you to meet."

"Okay," Kristen said hesitantly. By this point, she was a junior in high school and was following a good path. She wondered if her brother would try to lead her astray.

Kristen flew to California later that month. When Carson picked her up at the airport, she almost didn't recognize him. Standing before her was a clean-shaven young man in a nice pair of jeans and a collared shirt. Carson beamed across the airport at his sister with happiness.

When they arrived at his apartment, Kristen looked around with awe. "Wow, Carson, things sure seem to be different since the last time I talked to you."

Carson smiled. "That's why I wanted you to come visit me. Just a few months ago, I was down at a bar, using money I managed to scrape up on the streets to buy a few drinks and forget about the rejections I had been facing every day. There was this man, Preacher Robert. He came up to the bar and sat next to me and just started talking. Apparently he goes to bars and talks with people about their lives. Well, I told him I had hit rock bottom and that I didn't have a home, a job, nothing but the whiskey in the bottom of my glass." Carson said.

"What did he say?" Kristen asked.

"He said he wanted to help me. He took me in, helped me get my life together. He taught me how to accept the Lord as my savior. And it worked. I haven't touched any drugs since."

Kristen beamed at her brother. "That is wonderful, Carson!"

Carson held her hand. "I know we were never really into church, but you need to come to mine. I want you to meet Preacher Robert."

The next day, Kristen attended the service at Carson's church. When she saw the other members of the church wearing jeans and t-shirts, she was dumbfounded. This was nothing like the pomp and circumstance of her church back home. When she listened to Preacher Robert give his sermon, Kristen felt as if he was talking directly to her.

"Wow," Kristen whispered into Carson's ear. "It seems there's more to going to church than just Sunday service."

At the end of the service, Preacher Robert approached Kristen and Carson.

"Preacher Robert, this is my sister, Kristen," said Carson.

"Pleasure to meet you, Kristen," said Preacher Robert as he shook her hand. "Tell me Kristen, have you ever accepted the Lord as your savior."

"Not out loud," admitted Kristen.

"If you really want to live for the Lord, I'm going to lead you through a prayer."

Preacher Robert took Kristen to the front of the church. Along with a few of the church members, they recited a prayer. In that moment, Kristen felt as if an immense weight was being lifted off of her shoulders. The empty hole within her heart left by her father was filled instead by the Lord. At that moment, her life changed forever.

When Kristen returned home to Colorado, she told her mother how she had been saved. They found a nondenominational church similar to her brother's to attend and while at the service, her mother felt a strong, unfamiliar feeling. The same fire that burned within her children was now ignited in her as well.

Kristen wondered why the Lord hadn't entered their lives earlier, when they needed Him the most. She knew there must have been a reason why her family found God that year. From that moment on, Kristen knew she could get through anything in life and that she could walk down any path with a smile on her face.

Indeed, Kristen was right. A couple years later, while she was in college, her mother passed away. Kristen was heartbroken. Her mother was more than just her mother – she was also her father and her best friend. If it weren't for the Lord's presence in her life at this point in her journey, Kristen would have felt like an abandoned orphan.

"She's in a better place," her brother said during their mother's funeral, enveloping Kristen within his embrace.

Still living in Colorado, Kristen took solace in her family and her college sweetheart, Jacob. She was only too aware of the tragic marriage her mother had experienced with her father, but she was hopeful that things could be different with Jacob. He was a nice Christian man. When their college graduation arrived, Jacob told Kristen he wanted to move to Nashville to pursue his music career. Before he did though, he wanted Kristen to become his wife. She was ecstatic. Her brother had moved to Nashville the year before, so Kristen felt that getting married and moving to Music City would be the perfect way to surround herself with both her faith and family.

The very first thing Kristen did when she moved to Nashville was to find a new church. She knew that no matter what else was going on in her life, she wanted to always have the warm embrace of her church and her Lord around her. Her next step was developing a career. Throughout Kristen's life, her mother had been a sponsor of children with alcoholic parents and would help guide them through their troubling teenage years. Having seen her mother's dedication had ignited a passion to help teens and it felt right when she found a job as a social worker for teenagers in state custody. She saw herself in these teens and the person she could have been if she hadn't found God when she did. She saw how much pain her mother had suffered by marrying a man who had abandoned her and had succumbed to drugs and alcohol. Although she had never witnessed what a happy, true marriage was, Kristen felt she was living the real deal. At least, that's what she thought.

Five-and-a-half years into her marriage, Kristen made a shocking discovery about Jacob. A few months earlier, he had cheated on her with another woman. Kristen was devastated. She had uprooted her life to move to Nashville with Jacob and other than her brother, he was the only family she had. As hard as it was, Kristen knew she couldn't remain with someone who had broken the sanctity of marriage. Heartbroken and alone, she filed for divorce.

Kristen's church welcomed her with open arms. Without the continued and loving support of her pastor, her friends at church, her brother, and most importantly, God, Kristen would have broken down completely. She began to come to terms with the fact that she could be alone forever.

"You can't give up," Carson told her one cold day in December, mere weeks after her divorce was finalized. "You are going to find someone who will love and cherish you, in sickness and in health. God will ensure this."

During this time it was really the church and her community that sustained Kristen.

She could have traveled a very dark road but with the love of so many around her she was able to move forward. It very much reminded me of the good folks in Hillsboro who would always come together to support each other in the roughest times.

With great reluctance, Kristen joined an online dating site. She felt lost in the sea of eligible bachelors vying for her attention. How could she truly ever trust anyone again? The only man who interested her was a former semi pro-football player named Logan. He had messaged her a few months after she joined the site, noticing that they were both from the same hometown. "I noticed you moved from Colorado to Tennessee, which do you like better," he wrote.

Kristen responded to his message. To her surprise, Logan wasn't anything like she expected. Rather than trying to court her, Logan wanted to be her friend. For the next couple of years, Kristen and Logan remained solid pen pals. When her high school reunion approached, she knew they would finally have the chance to meet in person. She still felt her relationship with Logan was nothing more than a friendship. That is, until she returned to Colorado and met him. She ended up falling head over heels in love in only four days.

Logan was everything Kristen had always wanted in a man. A year after they first met in person, Kristen and Logan married, and he moved to Nashville to be with her. Life with Logan was nearly perfect. That didn't mean however, that they didn't have their heartbreaks. Just a year into their marriage, Logan lost his father to colon cancer and his mother to a tragic murder suicide. Because Kristen had walked through so much grief in her own life she felt that perhaps God was preparing her to help her husband walk through his own grief. Logan fell into a deep depression, but Kristen stayed by his side.

"I know exactly how you feel," Kristen would tell Logan.

Rather than creating a rift between them, the struggles they faced only made them stronger. Kristen knew that no matter what happened in the future, her bond with her husband was eternal.

One day, at a couple's conference, Kristen and Logan heard Pastor Jay speak. Pastor Jay was nothing like their current pastor. His energy and passion for the Lord was electric. "Logan," said Kristen, "I think it's time we start going to Pastor Jay's Church." They were welcomed to their new church with open arms. Its mission statement rang loud and clear – "Loving God, Servicing the World." Kristen became a young life leader at her church mentoring young teenage girls. She also began running her own small groups, and it was at one of these meetings where she met Heather. A newcomer to the church, Heather felt like an outsider.

"You should come over to my house for dinner," Kristen offered one day. Heather's eyes lit up. "I would love to."

Also at church, Kristen met an older woman named Mary. Ever since Kristen had lost her mother, she had prayed for a spiritual mom to take her place. A loving mother of three, Mary gladly filled that role. It may have taken 10 years for God to answer, but she knew God had brought Mary to her.

Kristen's life was finally coming together. The only bump in the road was a partial knee replacement she needed when she turned forty. Kristen knew that God would get her through the surgery. As she sat in her hospital bed, her hands to her chest with her head bowed in prayer, Kristen felt something strange on her chest. Her fingers caressed a large lump on the side of her breast. She thought it was nothing to worry about, but she brought it up to her doctor when he came in to see her.

"We'll get it checked out, just in case," he said. Behind his warm smile, Kristen noticed the fear in his voice. She began to expect the worse – and she was right. At the age of forty, Kristen was diagnosed with breast cancer.

"We caught it early," her doctor assured after he broke the news to her. "You will get through this." Unwaveringly she said, "I want to make sure I do, I want a double mastectomy."

Her doctor began explaining to her the next steps that she would have to take. Kristen would be subject to an endless number of hospital stays and chemotherapy sessions. She nodded stoically while her doctor talked to her and Logan, but the moment she and Logan got back to their car, she began sobbing. She felt overcome with a sense of fear and frailty she had never felt before. "God," she managed to utter between sobs as Logan held her in his arms, "I know you are trusting me with this journey. If you are giving me this challenge you probably want me to do something big. I will make sure that anybody and everybody who hears my story will not remain untouched by my faith. I want to give you the glory and the credit."

"Amen," whispered Logan, brushing back a strand of hair from his wife's face.

When Kristen returned home from her mastectomy, she felt as if she were a whole new person. Scars covered her chest and a long draining tube was inserted into the side of her chest. She worried how Logan would react to all the changes to her body, not to mention how helpless she had become. She already had one husband break their vows to her. Would Logan do the same?

"Honey, it's time to clean your wounds," Logan said before they went to bed. This was the moment that Kristen feared the most, even more than the mastectomy itself. As Logan began to undress and clean her wounds, he could feel Kristen tensing up. He looked up at Kristen.

"Honey, I'm fine. It's going to be okay. You are not alone."

Kristen began crying. "I'm sorry you have to experience this," she said.

He held Kristen's hands within his own. "This procedure saved your life. If I had to drain and clean your wounds every day for the rest of my life I would, because I love you and that was my commitment to you." He wiped Kristen's tears from her face.

The love that Kristen received from her husband was mirrored by her church and the other survivors who surrounded her with support. Church members would constantly call Kristen's home to check on her. When she became weak, they began to wash her hair and bring her meals. Still, the changes that were happening to Kristen's body were too much for her to bear. Every day after she went to chemo, she would find large clumps of her hair on her pillow.

Heather drove Kristen to her chemotherapy sessions because Kristen couldn't drive herself due to the medications. Heather packed lunch boxes with peppermints and dark chocolate for when Kristen became nauseous. The two passed time by playing card games and talking. Before long, Kristen began looking forward to her chemo sessions because it was a chance to have girl talk.

"God has a plan," Heather reminded Kristen as she brushed hair out of her face, only to have long locks remain in her hand. "He has it all under control." Heather pulled out a pink bandana from her purse and handed it to Kristen, who had tears in her eyes.

When Kristen went to church that Sunday, she wore the bandana that Heather gave her. To her surprise, she wasn't alone. Every member of her church was sporting a pink bandana, smiling at her when she walked in.

Logan, who stood by his wife's side, squeezed her hand. "See? I told you that you are not alone."

Kristen flew down the street, her pink bandana blowing in the wind. She never felt so free in her life. Several months had passed since her initial breast cancer diagnosis, and it had been five weeks since her last chemo appointment. With a new lease on life, Kristen joined a motorcycle riding club. Although she was still hesitant about her skills, she had promised herself that after her chemo was complete, she would live life to the fullest. Logan and Kristen were on their way to meet the rest of their motorcycle chapter at a local coffee shop. With Logan riding in front of her, Kristen felt unstoppable.

A block away from the coffee shop, Logan made a right turn, and Kristen went to follow. All of a sudden, Kristen's wheel hit a dip in the road. Her motorcycle lurched forward into a four-inch high median in the road. In an instant, Kristen was flying through the air across three lanes of traffic. Her bike fell with a loud bang onto the bumper of a stopped blue sedan, and Kristen fell to the ground with a sickening thud. With her legs spread out in front of her, Kristen sat in the middle of the road in shock.

The man in the blue sedan jumped out of his car and looked down at Kristen.

"Don't move a muscle! I'm calling 911."

Within a few minutes, the EMTs were at Kristen's side. Her legs throbbed with mind-numbing pain. "That's my wife, that's my wife!" Kristen saw Logan push through the crowd, looking pale. He crouched down next to her. "Honey, what happened?'

"I don't know, my legs hurt but I think I'm going to be fine," she assured him.

"We're going to lift you up," said one of the EMTs. He motioned to the other paramedics. "Let's do it, on the count of three, one... two...three!"

Kristen shrieked. Her vision became white as her entire body became throttled with an immense pain, greater than any she had ever felt before. She was carried to the ambulance, which sped off the moment she was safely inside.

Within a few minutes Kristen had arrived at Stone Crest Medical Center in Smyrna, just south of Nashville. As she was being wheeled into the emergency department a nurse with a glass of water and a pill came up to her. "You're going to need this," she said knowingly.

While Kristen was waiting for her x-rays to come back, Pastor Jay walked through the emergency room doors looking frazzled.

"Kristen, what happened? Are you okay?"

"I'm fine," she said wearily. "I just don't know how, or why."

Pastor Jay held her hand and nodded sympathetically, "Even though you are hurting, you need to trust in God."

"I know," she said. "He obviously has more plans for me. I could have died today and He saved me for a reason."

Kristen's doctor came back with her x-rays. "Your fracture is much worse than we thought," he told her. "We will need to send you to Vanderbilt Hospital."

It was 2 a.m. by the time Kristen arrived at Vanderbilt. She took off her bandana and while wiping the sweat off her head, she felt the tiny fuzz of hair that had begun growing in, and sighed. The victorious energy that was flowing through her veins just hours before had been substituted with pain and regret. I saw the pain on her face when I walked up to her, holding her x-ray. She was anxious and we talked about her injuries. We spent thirty minutes together and I explained how we would fix her leg. But with her other medical problems it was going to be a challenge to save her leg.

Kristen was one of my first trauma patients who had previously survived an extensive battle with cancer, and I knew I had to treat her with caution. Her bones were weaker and her body would be slower in healing with an increased chance for infection. Each time I met a patient with a history of cancer, I felt very connected because of my dad's fight with the same disease process. Seeing Kristen brought back so many memories of my father and his losing battle with liver cancer. He had fought until the very end, but in the last days of his life we had spent some of our most precious time together, time of which I will always be thankful. When I talked with Kristen, somehow I just knew that she would end up surprising me. I explained to her that we would start by putting a metal frame on her leg and then address the break when her swelling went down and when the risk of infection was lower.

Kristen didn't sleep for a minute that night. With Logan snuggled up in her bed next to her, Kristen replayed that moment on her bike over and over. She knew she needed to trust in God, but she still couldn't understand how everything had changed for her in one split second. Why her, for the second time in a year?

Later that morning, I performed surgery on Kristen's right leg. I cleaned her wounds and put on an external fixator. The surgery went perfectly. I met Logan right after the surgery and updated him on her condition.

For the next week while Kristen was in the hospital, Logan worked overtime at a car dealership. When he returned home in the morning, he would sleep for a few hours before heading over to visit Kristen.

"Honey, you must be so tired. You should just come and visit me every other day," she insisted.

"I can't leave you," he responded, tears in his eyes. "I wish it was me in that hospital bed instead of you."

Logan's devotion to Kristen and the love and care he provided was one of the most important factors in determining how she would do. As a surgeon I have seen the power of love do amazing things and help people recover when many people believed they couldn't. In my own family as a small child I had watched my mother stay by my father's bedside in hospital after hospital as he battled chronic illness – she would never leave him even for a minute and I believe this made all the difference.

Kristen was discharged to a skilled nursing facility while she healed before her second surgery. While she recovered, Kristen listened to a radio worship station. The prayers helped her get through the long days while Logan rested at home. On the night of their twelfth anniversary, Logan surprised her with takeout Chinese food.

"Happy anniversary, honey," he said with a smile.

Kristen's eyes welled up with tears. "Happy anniversary."

Logan took her to dinner that night. He pushed her in a wheel chair to the dining room where they enjoyed their dinner together. It wasn't a typical, romantic night out, but it was perfect. Kristen returned to Vanderbilt ten days later for her second surgery.

"Don't worry," I reassured her before heading into the operating room. "Everything is going to be fine. You must keep the faith."

Kristen nodded. "I will."

In the operating room, I removed the external fixator I had put in a few weeks earlier and replaced it with plates and screws. These plates would hold her bones together and help them heal over time. When Kristen woke later that day she felt immense pain in her legs.

"I would rather have a double mastectomy twice than have to do that again," Kristen told Logan, who was sitting attentively at her side. Logan looked at his wife with worry. "There's something I have to tell you," he said.

Two months earlier, Logan had been injured in an accident while on the job but he did not tell Kristen at the time. He knew he would eventually need to get surgery once all the paperwork had been filed and unfortunately that time had now come. He reached over and held her hand, "Don't worry honey," Logan reassured her, "If it ends up happening, we will find a way to get through it."

For the next few weeks while still in the hospital, Kristen was full of anxiety. To her relief, however, Logan was able to stay at her side. Before Kristen was released, a physical therapist came to help her get back on her feet. When Kristen stood for the first time, she felt a jolt of pain in her left knee, the leg that had not been broken.

"Something's wrong, I know it," she said. When I heard what had happened, I ordered a CAT scan. Indeed, we had missed seeing a small hairline fracture in Kristen's left knee, the one that had been replaced several years prior to the accident. This really complicated things for her as now she couldn't walk on either leg.

When I told her the news, it took all of Kristen's strength to keep from crying. Still, it wasn't until the next day, when Logan took Kristen home that she truly realized the massive trauma she had sustained and how close she was to never stepping foot in her house again. She wondered why this had happened to her. She already had overcome breast cancer; she wasn't even finished with her radiation therapy.

"Austin from our church and Justin from our motorcycle chapter helped build this ramp for us," Logan told her as he pushed the wheelchair toward the house.

As soon as Logan opened the door, their dogs came running up to Kristen. As they jumped up on her lap and celebrated her return, tears formed in Kristen's eyes. The couple had decided earlier in the year before she was diagnosed with breast cancer that they wanted to have children, but once she was diagnosed, they realized they would have to wait at least another year. Now how much longer would she have to wait? Would her family forever consist of her and Logan and their dogs, or was there a baby in their future? Kristen knew it was by God's Grace she was able to return to her house with her loving husband. She knew He was keeping her alive for a reason; maybe one of those reasons was a child.

She remained bed-ridden for the next six weeks and was constantly reminded of God's presence in her life. During this time, she received an outpouring of love from members of her church who took turns coming over and making dinner. Heather was always just a phone call away and of course, her greatest support was Logan. Every day when he came home from work he would sit at Kristen's side in the armchair he had set up next to her hospital bed in the living room.

Six weeks later Kristen was doing very well and I started letting her put weight on the right side and she was relieved. In addition to the helplessness she felt lying in bed all day, Logan's impending surgery still weighed on her mind. They still hadn't heard any more details about when his surgery would be scheduled. Kristen was terrified of what would happen if Logan had his surgery while she was still in her wheelchair. Who would get her up the ramp and into her home? Heather, even with her big heart and never-ending support, was too small to thrust her up the ramp in her chair. She once again began to become overcome with anxiety.

"Just pray," Heather told her soothingly one night while she made Kristen and Logan dinner. "God will take care of everything."

"I have," Kristen replied. "Every night I listen to my worship station to get me through the night. Still, I ask God why I have to go through this. Why Logan has to go through this."

Logan squeezed her hand. "I think it's time we go back to church."

"I think so too," Kristen whispered.

That Sunday, Kristen woke up bright and early. With Logan's help, she got dressed and ready to head to church for the first time since her accident. She felt butterflies in her stomach. She was aching to go back, but she wondered what it would be like to sit in the back in her wheelchair and listen to her pastor speak again.

When they reached the grand doors of the church and Logan swung open the door, Kristen felt a sense of peace overcome her body. As he rolled her down the aisle to the edge of the last pew, church members turned to look at her. The love and warmth in their eyes calmed Kristen's soul. Tears welled up in her eyes.

For the next few hours, she was surrounded by her friends from church. They huddled around her, telling her they were praying for her recovery and keeping her in their thoughts.

Matthew, one of the associate pastors, sat next to Kristen and looked at her with awe. "You know I love God, Kristen, but if I were in your shoes, I wouldn't be able to handle it as well as you."

In that moment, Kristen comprehended the strength that she had shown throughout all of her experiences. The strength she showed dealing with her alcoholic father, her cancer, her motorcycle accident and the resulting trauma didn't come from her, but from God. He had been watching over her since she was a little girl, sitting in her grandmother's lap, hoping for a father to love and protect her. Little did she know, she already had a Father.

A few months later, Logan's surgery was finally scheduled. The week before his surgery, Kristen came to see me again.

"You never cease to amaze me, Kristen," I said. "You've continued to heal quickly. You are ready to begin walking again, with a walker."

Kristen squealed with delight. It was perfect timing, because that meant she would be back on her feet when Logan would be in the hospital recovering.

Kristen still needed to receive her final treatments of radiation therapy which had been delayed due to her accident, but were required to ensure that her cancer would stay in remission. While Logan was in the hospital for his surgery, Kristen walked from her house to the clinic with her walker. Once there, the radiation therapy drained her energy, leaving her feeling tired and lifeless. The walk back felt as if it was a never-ending journey. Logan was only going to be in the hospital for a few days, but that meant Kristen would have to make the same trip by herself a second time. Her legs burning with agonizing pain, she felt as if she were about to collapse on her walk back to her house. When she finally reached the door and pushed it open. She almost fell over with surprise. There, at the kitchen counter, stood Logan, his arm in a sling. He turned when he saw Kristen, holding up a spatula.

"Hi honey, I was discharged early today." he said with a warm smile. "I'm making dinner."

Kristen cried with happiness. As they sat at the table enjoying their dinner, chicken fingers and French fries, Logan reached over and caressed Kristen's hand. "Isn't your brother performing at Twelfth and Porter (a popular club in Nashville) next weekend?"

"Yes, he is," said Kristen excitedly. "We should go."

That weekend, Logan, Kristen, and Heather headed out to watch her brother perform. As Logan pushed Kristen up a hill toward the door of the club that night, she felt an unconditional love for her husband. She knew that no matter what, he would always be there to support her, pushing her up the next mountain of troubles they had to face.

Soon, Kristen was able to go back to work. She made sure to keep her leg propped up, as she was told to do, while at home and in the office. By the end of January, she was able to begin walking on a walking boot. She was ecstatic. She began to feel pain in her leg when she walked, but she shrugged it off. Of course it would take some time to adjust. When two weeks passed, and the pain subsisted, she asked her physical therapist, Sandra if she should be worried.

"Is it supposed to hurt like this?" She asked Sandra.

"It's probably your muscles trying to adjust," Sandra responded.

When her leg began to swell, Kristen knew that something was very wrong. During her breast cancer surgery, she had to have some of her lymph vessels removed, which made her susceptible to lymphedema in her legs. She made an appointment to see me.

"Did it hurt when you walked in just now?" I asked her when she came into the clinic room.

"Yes," she replied. "It's been getting worse."

"I'm going to order some x-rays," I said. "Don't worry, everything will be fine," I assured her before I left the room.

Ten minutes later, I came back with her results. "Well, Kristen," I began, "I have good news and bad news."

Kristen took a deep breath. "Tell me the good news first," she said.

"The good news is that your bone is starting to fuse, which means your leg is healing. The bad news is that you've broken all your hardware."

Kristen looked over at Logan. She couldn't help but laugh. "I've barely walked anywhere! How could this have happened?" We talked and I explained that we could still try and heal her without surgery and with a small device called a bone stimulator. While it was a long shot, it was worth a try.

When she went home that night, she began her new treatment and over the next few weeks, she began a new routine. After dinner, she would lie in bed and would turn on her bone stimulator, closing her eyes while she listened to her worship station. As she listened to the pastor over the radio, she felt herself healing not only physically, but spiritually. The challenges she had faced in her life were more than she ever could have expected. She wondered if she would be sitting here today, if Carson had never entered that bar decades ago. The pastor who had approached him not only changed her brother's life, but had saved hers in the process. Without God, she would have given up a long time ago. Kristen knew that God had channeled his power to help her through several important people in her life – the members of her church, her doctors, and her loving husband. Since his accident, Logan had numerous permanent restrictions that prevented him from performing the physical tasks that he used to do easily. Because of this, he was released from his job and was unable to find another one. Despite the stress that he now faced, his love for Kristen never faltered.

Eight weeks later, she returned to my office. I examined her leg and looked up at her with a smile. Despite her cancer and broken plates and screws, she had healed.

Logan turned to Kristen, embracing her in his arms and kissing her on her forehead.

"Thank you, Dr. Sethi," Kristen said with happiness. "I felt as if this day would never come." Kristen had been through so much and if one were to consider the basic facts including her history of cancer and the severe nature of her injury, most would have predicted a very bad end result. Somehow Kristen was able rise above it all and get back on her feet, even with the odds against her. I very much believe that she had the powerful combination of faith, family, and community that allowed her to heal and reach beyond herself. As I sat there in my clinic talking with her I could not help but think about the same powerful forces that have guided me and made me who I am.

The past year of Kristen's life had been a blur. Despite all their troubles, Kristen and Logan's love grew even stronger. Before she knew it, their thirteenth wedding anniversary had arrived. Although they were tight on money, they had received a gift card to a romantic restaurant they were saving for their special day.

As Kristen sat across from Logan at the restaurant during their anniversary dinner, she couldn't help but feel conscious of the brace on her leg.

"I feel as if we celebrate our marriage every day," she told him. "We didn't have to come out today. Not a day goes by that I don't thank God for having you at my side."

"I feel the same way," Logan said. "But still, think of how far we have come. At this time last year, we were in the nursing home, sitting in the dining room with our Chinese takeout."

Kristen laughed. "Yes, I remember. It feels like just yesterday."

"But it wasn't. You have come such a long way since then."

"You're right," Kristen replied. "Sometimes the challenges seem never-ending. But God is ensuring that I will live through them. These are two anniversaries that could have easily passed me by."

Logan reached over the table and held Kristen's hands within his own. "But they didn't," he reminded her with a loving smile. "And there will always be more anniversaries to come."

Not long after that celebration, Kristen had surgery to remove the broken metal in her leg. The surgery went well, and recovery seemed to be going well. However, six weeks after the surgery, the bottom of her incision was healing slowly, and her leg was red. She contacted me and sent photos of her leg. I then told her to get into my office right away, because she was sicker than she thought she was, and that I would have to admit her to the hospital and do emergency surgery that afternoon. She came in and as I looked at her leg, I confirmed it was infected and I would have to do surgery. The infection had also traveled to her radiated side of her chest, and her breast implant would have to be removed by one of my colleagues.

As Kristen sat waiting to go back for surgery, she looked at Logan and said, "My life was almost taken from me last year TWICE, and now this threat to my life? The only thing that will happen is God will get more glory in my story through this next bump in the road." Both surgeries went well, and the infection wasn't as bad as we thought it would be once we got in there. Kristen spent five days in the hospital as the infectious disease team of doctors tried to figure out what type of infection it was. It turns out it was a Staph infection, which very much could have threatened her life. Once again, while in the hospital, trying to figure out why she was going through yet another major trial with her health, she would listen to a worship station on the radio to soothe her soul. She turned to God for peace, and for strength to get through yet another hard time in her life. She was facing months of antibiotics, a lot of follow-up appointments and more reconstruction surgery on her chest. Eventually over the next few months, as she had done every single time, Kristen beat the odds and continued to heal. She started to walk without help and once again, Logan was by her side every day, loving her so well through yet another trial.

Together they drew closer to God and to each other, and were embraced by the warmth of their close friends and church family as they moved forward to face the next life challenge much stronger from the difficulties they had already endured.

Progress Notes on Kristen

Kristen underwent reconstructive surgery on her chest about two years after her original breast cancer diagnosis. With the help of her loving husband, friends, and church, she will undergo her final reconstructive surgery and another knee replacement in the coming months. She recently attended the National Women's Survivor Convention for cancer survivors that takes place every year in Nashville. There, she had the privilege to meet other women who underwent a similar journey as her own. She continues to believe in living life to the fullest and relies on her faith in God to keep her going. Recently together with Logan, she adopted her first child.

Susan

It is commonly believed that immediately before a near-death experience, a person's life flashes before one's eyes. That didn't happen to Susan. One moment she was sitting at a red light on the way to her father's annual Memorial Day cookout with her family, and the next she was waking up in the hospital, wondering where she was and how she got there. If she did have her whole life flash before her eyes in the few minutes before the oncoming car slammed into her, she would have seen the rolling countryside of Columbia, Tennessee.

Susan grew up in this small town in a single family home with her half-sister Amy and her two brothers, Dylan, and Rick. Her father left when she was still young and was absent for most of her life. Susan and I share the values of growing up in a small town in Tennessee and much like I had, she learned the power of faith, family, and community at a very early age.

Her mother was her best friend. Whenever she or her siblings got into trouble or needed advice, they would talk to their understanding mom, who would never talk down to anyone. Her mother always made it clear that neither she nor any other female should ever be dependent on anyone else. Her mom would always say "you work hard to get what you get in life. You never take from someone else." Her mother's advice was heard and obeyed because the only person who Susan ever depended upon was herself and God to carry her through. Perhaps that's why Susan's life-long dream was to open up her own business, a real estate company, so she could feel the pride in being able to support herself.

Every week at church she prayed for that dream. At Friendship Missionary Baptist Church, they were all one big family and Susan would spend several days each week surrounded by the warmth of that family, listening to her minister as he shared God's messages or by singing His praises in the choir. To Susan, her family and her faith meant everything. Still, she felt as if her life in Columbia was just not moving fast enough. If she were to live the dream of owning her own business within the next 10 years, she would have to make a bold move soon.

Upon graduation from college, she decided to move to Atlanta, Georgia where she began her first job at a fast food chain. Once she became accustomed to working in customer service, she moved up the ranks and began working in accounting at a large supermarket chain where she learned the ins and outs of running a large business. These were vital skills she would use in the future when she was ready to create Mill's Realty, which would be dedicated to her mom Caroline Mills, who inspired her to envision grand dreams and a trust in God to make them come true.

Susan spent three years in Atlanta, cherishing her independence and her new life in the big city. When she came home from work one Friday, Susan called her mother to tell her about her week. When her mother picked up the phone, her voice was quivering. Her doctor had just told her that she had cancer. I understand the power of a phone call like this as I had received a similar call about my father in 2003. My life would never be the same and the same would hold true for Susan.

During the next few months, Susan's life was a whirlwind. Her mother had late stage cancer of both her breast and lung. What followed were months of chemotherapy and going in and out of remission. In addition to the stress of her mother's illness, Susan found out her sister Amy, still in high school, was pregnant. Susan wasn't prepared for the dramatic changes that were happening. Her younger siblings would be left alone without a mother and the only other family they had other than Susan, was their church. Her minister and friends provided their never-ending love, support, and prayers during her mother's illness. Susan moved back home to take care of her family, while her mother's condition worsened with each passing day.

Columbia had changed very little since she left. To Susan, life in the small town couldn't compare to the life that she had built in the big city. She missed Atlanta. She wondered if this was the plan God had for her, so different from the one that she had envisioned.

A few months later, Amy had her child and a few weeks after that, her mother passed away. Susan was only twenty-three years old. Losing her best friend and mother was too much for her, but once again, her church was there to console her. Members of the clergy stepped up and over the next few years would help raise her brothers and sisters as if they were their own children. Her minister was quick to remind her that her mother, just like her grandmother, would always be watching over her, especially in moments when she needed them the most.

With her church's support in raising her siblings, Susan was able to move back to Atlanta where she returned to her previous job and soon was happy and content again. She loved her job and enjoyed working directly with customers. She could wear jeans to work, had great perks, received good health insurance, and was paid every Friday. To Susan, being able to support herself meant everything. She continued attending church and Bible study every Sunday and on Saturdays she helped with the children's choir.

Susan remained in Atlanta for the next 10 years all while working her way up at her job. One night while she was out with her friends, she noticed a young man watching her from across the dance floor. It didn't take him long to approach her, introduce himself as Larry, and asked her to dance. She was immediately charmed. Larry was self-employed, which meant he had the freedom to travel and live his life the way he wanted. They spent the rest of the night dancing and sharing their life stories. Within a few hours she envisioned her future with him. They would get married and have kids and build their own lives together in the excitement of the big city that allowed her to dream of the future she always wanted.

Larry and Susan began to date, and over the next few months their relationship blossomed. She had never been in love before, but she found it here and she knew this was the eternal bond between a man and a woman that they talked about in church.

While she lived in Atlanta, her siblings, Amy, Dylan, and Rick grew up, got married, and started their own families. Although she was far away from home, her family's bond remained strong. Every month, Amy would visit Susan for a girl's night out that she always looked forward to, but sadly, it would always remind her of how much she missed the rest of her family back in Tennessee. Even though she felt lonely living on her own, Susan's faith and desire for independence kept her from moving in with Larry.

"Not before marriage," she would remind him every time he asked. One day, he finally got the hint. He grasped her hand, got down on one knee and opened up a small velvet box, within which was the diamond ring that would adorn her hand for the rest of her life.

Susan was happier than she had ever been. They planned the wedding for the following April 27, which was also her birthday. Once married, she and Larry would live together and start their new family in Atlanta. Susan felt her life was headed in the right direction.

Out of the blue one day, Susan was surprised when her father, Russell, called. She hadn't heard from him in years. He said he wanted to be a part of her life and prove to her that his previous abandonment was a mistake that he would never make again. She was his only daughter and he wanted her close to him. She was torn. Her family meant everything to her, and if there was one single thing that defined her, it was putting her family's happiness first, even before her own. Her family was the one thing that was missing from her life in Atlanta. How could she deny her father the chance to have his? She had already lost one parent, maybe God had sent her another so that she could have someone to walk her down the aisle and to help raise his grandkids.

Although it was hard to leave Larry, Susan made the decision to move back to Tennessee that summer to be with her family. Larry promised that they would remain together during their time apart and assured her that he still wanted to marry her the following April as planned.

It felt weird to Susan to go back to Columbia after all this time. She knew her life would change when she moved back, but there was no way she could have expected what happened next. A month after Susan arrived back in Tennessee; she was looking forward to attending her father's Memorial Day cookout. Every year, he hosted the cookout at her aunt's house in Columbia. Her aunt didn't have any grandkids and loved for everyone to bring their families and enjoy a day of food, swimming, and family.

On the day of the cookout, Susan's Aunt Lana and cousin had come to pick up Susan, Amy, and Amy's daughter. As they always had done growing up, she and Amy began to argue over which side of the car they were going to sit. Although it was just a silly argument, this time, the outcome would end up deciding whose life was about to change forever.

Susan sat behind the driver's seat, so anxious about seeing her family and going back to Columbia that she forgot to buckle her seatbelt. Her brother Dylan and his family were in the car in front and Aunt Lana followed closely behind. Their plan was to follow each other out of the neighborhood and down Murfreesboro Road. A few minutes away from their home the car in which Susan was riding stopped at a red light. The light changed to green, a loud and thunderous crash occurred and for Susan, everything went black.

She awoke in an unfamiliar room. She saw tubes coming out of her arms and saw that she was hooked to a machine. She grasped the tubes and began to pull, trying to scream for help. She couldn't open her mouth, and suddenly an immense pain shot across her body. She felt confused and weak and drifted back to sleep. The next few days were the same. She would wake and try to free herself from the bed, wondering why she was there and how she got there. One time, she woke to find her arms restrained at her sides. There was a woman peering down at her. "Do you know where you are?" Her voice sounded as if she were standing at the end of a long tunnel.

"No," Susan said, drifting in and out of consciousness.

The woman looked worried. "Could you give me a thumbs up?" She asked. Susan tried to lift her thumb. Miraculously, she could. The woman smiled.

Susan soon realized this woman was her nurse. Every day her nurse came in and asked in the same soothing voice, "Do you know where you are?" Susan would shake her head no, and the nurse would reply, "You are at Vanderbilt Medical Center." This went on for several days before Susan was finally stable enough to remember her conversations with her nurse.

Soon, her entire family – her brothers and sisters, her Aunt Lana and cousin, her father, and Larry were allowed to visit. When she saw them, she tried to smile to show how happy she was to know they were all okay, but even that little movement caused pain to ripple through her body.

It was a week before Susan was able to put together the pieces of what had happened. Seconds after the light turned green and her

Aunt Lana started through the intersection, another car approaching from the other direction slammed into their car. Her niece flew out of the car and onto the street. Susan suffered the brunt of the blow, saving Amy from the high impact that crushed the vehicle. The nurses told her that she was unconscious in the car for more than twenty minutes as emergency responders tried to get her out of the burning vehicle. She was severely injured, suffering fractures to her pelvis, her ribs, and her clavicle. Her lungs had collapsed and her aorta was injured. Susan had several surgeries to fix her injuries, including the one I performed to stabilize her pelvis in the days immediately following the accident. Her sister Amy had suffered her own injuries and was taken to another hospital closer to where she was injured. However, she refused treatment at that hospital so she could rush to Vanderbilt Medical Center and check on Susan and her daughter. It wasn't until she knew they were both alive that she allowed herself to be treated.

Amy, Aunt Lana and their daughters were released from medical care a few days after the accident, leaving Susan as the only family still in the hospital. When she heard about the accident and how she had sustained her injuries, she thanked not only God, but her mother and grandmother. She knew that her minister was right and that they must have been there to protect her. When she thought of her mother, she remembered what she had told her about the importance of having strength and trusting in God in times of struggle. This was the greatest struggle she had ever faced.

Beyond the physical suffering she faced, Susan hated being bed-ridden. She was used to working, moving around, and being a productive member of society. Becoming dependent on nurses just to go to the bathroom and on her family to provide her company as she lay imprisoned in her hospital bed was nearly unbearable. This was not the way her mother had raised her to live. The only thing keeping Susan sane during this time was her family and Larry. Although Larry wanted to be with her every day while she was in the hospital, he had to return to his work in Atlanta. Her father and Aunt Lana started taking turns staying with her. Her dad would be there for four days, and her aunt would be there the other three. She thought of what her dad had said to her when he first reached out to her the previous year, promising that no matter what, he would never leave her again.

After a few days, Susan started to become accustomed to her life at the hospital, at least as much as one can under these circumstances. The nurses would tell her she was the best patient they ever had. She took her medications without any fuss and she began recognizing me and her other doctors, thanking us often for saving her life nearly a month earlier. She asked me what she could do to get better faster. Unfortunately, the recovery process for someone who suffered a near-death accident like Susan was painfully long. There was nothing more Susan wanted than to get out of bed, and she would do anything to do it. Little did she realize what a challenge she would be facing for a long time.

One morning, she began throwing up. Everything she ate would only stay down for a few hours, and she would keel over in pain every time. It left her exhausted. A few hours later, Susan was throwing up again, this time uncontrollably. It was time for Plan B. Her nurse inserted a tube through her nose and down into her stomach to help ease the nausea. The tube was torture, and it didn't work, plus it caused Susan to begin bleeding from her nose and to cough and gag, gasping for air.

After four attempts to make the tube work, Susan cried out. "Stop, I can't take it anymore!" She pulled out the tube, covered in her own blood.

Her father was standing in the corner watching the incident. "I'm sorry," he said, "I can't watch this." He left the room but returned once the nurse had left. This was Susan's lowest point since arriving at the hospital. She tried to keep a brave face, to have faith in God and stay true to her mother, but she finally began to wonder "why me?" Susan was a good person. More than just feeling sorry for herself, she wondered how God could have done this to her family, who stayed by her side faithfully.

Susan had reached her darkest hour as her hope started to fade. From my own life experiences and caring for patients, I came to realize that what happened in these "moments" made all the difference and guided how one would move forward; would Susan fight or give up?

By now, the only thing that comforted her was being able to see her nieces and nephews. She hadn't been able to see them earlier in her stay because children were not allowed in the ICU. Now that she had been taken off the machines and moved into a regular room, they were allowed to finally come and visit.

Susan stayed in her new room for a few more weeks. Afterward, she was discharged from the hospital and moved to rehabilitation at Vanderbilt's Stallworth facility. She was determined to start walking as soon as she could, but she knew the odds were against her. The injuries she suffered were of the most dangerous kind and she was lucky to be alive. I told her it would take months for her to get back on her feet and walk again. That wasn't fast enough for Susan. Every day, she would get out of bed and place her feet on the floor, feeling excruciating pain shoot through her body every time she put any weight on her legs. Instead of listening to her body begging her to stop, she prayed. On other days, she cried. It took a lot to make Susan cry, but when she worked up to eight hours a day trying to get back to normal with no success, she cried.

One day, a man with a warm smile knocked on her door. He introduced himself and said he was from her church. He began to visit her several days a week and would sit with her after she had finished her rehab for the day. Even though it was hard for Susan to admit, she told him she was having trouble with her faith. He smiled and said he understood. She began to pour out all her feelings about everything that had occurred, wondering why it all happened to her, a faithful child of God. He listened calmly, and then responded. "Everything happens for a reason, it's all part of God's plan." He sounded just like her mother. He gave her confidence in her strength and in God's constant presence in her life.

After a few weeks of rehabilitation at Stallworth, Susan was discharged. Although she was relieved to be able to return home, everything just seemed to get worse. Her family had changed their entire schedules so they could have shifts to watch her. Amy would arrive around 4 a.m. and stay until 1 p.m. At that point, Dylan would come in and stay until 10 p.m. Her cousin would also stop by during the day to take care of her. Every day someone would come and cook for her, help her bathe, and would help her change her position in bed. Susan felt helpless. In order to help lighten up her mood, one day Amy offered to get her out of the house and take her shopping at Opry Mills.

"There's no way I'm going there in my wheelchair," Susan said determinedly. "I'll take the walker." That walk around the mall was the hardest thing she had ever done in her life. She felt like everyone was staring at her, and the pain that shot through her legs with every step made her want to fall to the ground and give up. Still, that walk with the walker meant so much to her because it proved that soon she might be able to walk on her own. She was on a strict deadline, April 27, the date she was to marry Larry, was only a few months away. That walk down the aisle was something she had dreamed of all her life, and she was going to do it no matter what.

As Susan was slowly improving, the medical bills from her treatment began to accumulate. She gave Amy her pin number for her retirement account, which she used to pay as much of her bills as she could. She also began to sell some of her most prized possessions, goods that she had worked hard to acquire, including her car. Her life savings, which she had planned to use to build a home with Larry in Atlanta, began to wither away. Amy suggested that she file for disability.

"No," Susan said adamantly, "I don't want to depend on the system to get me out of this. I'm going to depend on myself and God."

It soon got to the point that Susan couldn't afford to pay her rent, electricity, or water. If she broke her lease, she would have to pay even more. Her family began to help her out. Amy paid her cell phone bills so she could continue to talk to Larry every night while he remained in Atlanta. During their nightly conversations, they continued to plan for their wedding. Susan began to have the sinking feeling that she wouldn't be fully recovered in time to walk down the aisle, but she decided to wait and see how she progressed before sharing her fears with Larry. She also hated being so financially dependent on her family, so she decided to go ahead and file for unemployment and disability. After being denied several times, she became angry. She had a loving and supportive family, but she wondered what would other people do who were denied assistance and didn't have the same support? She was truly stranded. When her lease was up in February and she was still not able to walk on her own, there was no choice but to move in with Amy.

"Go ahead and go to work at your usual time," she told Amy, "I will get the kids ready for school and start making my own lunch."

Amy was hesitant about leaving Susan on her own because she knew it was still a struggle for her to get out of bed, much less get the kids up. Amy left her small lunch packs, the kind prepared for school children, for her to eat during the day. Even that was difficult for Susan, who could only use one arm effectively. Later that month, she came in for another surgery for her clavicle fracture, which was not healing properly. The surgery was another reminder that she was still a long way from recovery.

Susan's birthday and her wedding day were only a few weeks away. Still, she could not walk on her own. "I'm not walking down the aisle on a walker!" she said to Larry. He tried to convince her otherwise. Larry desperately wanted to marry Susan on April 27, like they had planned, but she was still refusing to move in with him in Atlanta until they were married. Since she didn't have enough money to move back to Atlanta and get a place of her own, this meant they had to maintain a long-distance romance during the time she needed him the most. She just hoped that he wouldn't give up on her.

"I'm going to stand up and walk for myself," she said with determination. "I really want to marry you on April 27, but I can't until I can walk on my own again. I promise you, though, once I start earning money again we are going to get married," she said. Larry knew Susan was worth the wait, so he agreed to postpone the wedding until she was fully recovered. However, Susan knew that learning how to walk was easier said than done. She began to fall into a deep depression. Every time she would watch shows on TV of people getting married and being happy, she began to cry. Every night, she had to call out to her cousin to help roll her from one side of the bed to the other. She didn't want to wake her cousin during the night to help her go to the bathroom, so she learned how to use a bedpan. Susan felt helpless. She wouldn't wish this life on her worst enemy.

A few weeks before her birthday, Susan began going to church again with Amy. As soon as she entered through those doors, she began to feel a little bit better.

"Susan!" cried Mrs. Griffin, one of her friends from church. She grabbed her arm with excitement. "It's great to have you back!"

"Thank you," she said quietly. All of a sudden she welled up with emotion. She hadn't realized how difficult it would be to go back to church and she remembered all the days she had missed; recalling all the missed Sunday school lessons and all the Saturday choir practices made her cry. Instead of going back to church again after that one Sunday, she began to watch the services on her church's website. It felt good to be a part of the service again, even though she wasn't ready to go in person.

On April 27, Susan lay in her bed and thought about what it would have been like to be in a white wedding dress that day, being showered with love from her friends and family. It had promised to be the most important day of her life. Amy, picking up on her sister's sadness, suggested they go out to eat and celebrate her birthday. She wasn't in the mood, but she agreed just to make Amy happy. After helping her into the car, Amy drove to a nearby restaurant. It was a big ordeal to get her out of the car and through the restaurant doors. Susan wondered if the trip was worth the pain and the sorrow.

"Surprise!"

Susan stood in shock as she gazed out at her entire family. They all stood with big smiles on their faces, smiling and clapping. She began to cry. These were not tears of joy, but of pain. Why did they surprise her like that? Why did they keep going out of their way to do things for her, reminding her how helpless she really was?

Susan was determined to reclaim her life and move forward. In my clinic, she would talk of the troubles she had been facing and I encouraged her to stay in faith and to trust in her family that had been so supportive throughout her struggle to live.

It was so difficult to watch patients like Susan face such adversity, to see them cry in pain and anguish. In these moments I just wanted to reach out and make it better and to be there as my father had done so many times for his patients in that small Manchester clinic.

Susan didn't know what to do. She decided to turn to God. "God," she said that night, while she lay in bed, "if you allow me to go back to work and start getting on my feet, I will get myself to church and I promise to be there every Sunday."

More than anything, Susan wanted to not be dependent on her family and be able to work again and participate in her church. She knew her mother would not be happy to know that she was acting so helpless. She was determined to do anything she could to get back on her feet.

In her effort to heal better and quicker, she began cutting down on her meals and going for a walk while her sister was at work every day. Being overweight put her at a higher risk of developing complications, so she worked hard to get back in shape. While walking, she prayed to God and looked to Him for help. With every step, she realized her life was not yet over. Instead, a new chapter was just beginning, and it was up to her to decide what to do with it. She couldn't change what had happened, but she could do things differently from this point forward.

Susan imagined what her headstone would have said if she had died at that moment. "Susan Grover, faithful to her friends and family, she died trying." Was that really who she was? Someone who always tried, but never succeeded? She decided to take the challenge God had given her and push forward.

She began to remember all the previous dreams and aspirations she had abandoned, and started figuring out how she could now achieve them. She wanted a family. If she couldn't do so because of her age, she would adopt. She wanted to get her real estate license and start her own business so she could be a provider for her family. She also wanted to pay back her family for all the help they had given her. More than anything, she wanted to start working again and buy herself a new car so she could go to church every Sunday and join the choir again, to fulfill her promise to God. When she did start earning money again, she figured, she wouldn't penny pinch anymore but spend it on things she wanted. She knew now that life was precious and could be gone in a split second. It was time for her to live her life the way it was supposed to be lived.

She remembered the lessons that her pastor had reiterated almost every week while she watched the service online. During that time, it seemed he was talking directly to her, as if he knew exactly what she needed to know from God. It seemed he deliberately reminded her of the message every week until it reverberated inside of her. "If you admit your mistakes and your faults," he would begin, "God will accept your apology, and he will bless you."

Susan knew it was a mistake to question her faith. If it weren't for God, she would never have had the strength to continue her life. As she returned to her house after a short walk one day, she stopped outside her door and talked to God. "I'm sorry for ever questioning you, and the existence of your constant presence in my life. Everything you do has a purpose, and I promise that I will get my life back in order."

From that moment on, Susan decided that she needed to make some major changes. She continued to pray and think about the new direction in her life over the next few weeks. She eventually came to the decision that she wanted to leave her position at the supermarket where she had worked for 10 years. She loved working there, but it was time to make a change and find a new job that gave her a sense of meaning and purpose. However she knew all that had to wait because she still wasn't able to live on her own and she still relied on her sister and her family for help. Until she was completely independent again, she didn't want to marry Larry and become a burden for her new husband. She knew Larry loved her enough to wait for her until she was ready. Although it was tough to continue to put her life with Larry on hold, Susan decided she would stay in Tennessee with her family until she was fully recovered. Since she would continue to live at her sister's house, she began to look for a new job close to the neighborhood. After a few more weeks of searching, she found a position working as a mid-day assistant at a nearby pre-school.

Working at the preschool ended up being very tough on her. All of the children had special needs and they bit, kicked, and fought with her every day. Most of them couldn't speak and she couldn't understand what they wanted. When she came home from work, she was exhausted and in pain. Having weaned herself off her prescription pain killers and medications, she now took only Tylenol, and patiently waited as the pain slowly ebbed away. Her work was hard, but she loved the kids too much to leave. She began jogging to help her lose weight. Throughout this time, Susan continued to visit me in clinic every few weeks so I could check on her. Her father was at her side every time. I was impressed with her progress and noticed that she looked stronger and more energized with every visit.

Susan became acclimated to her new job at the preschool over time. However, she continued to dream of owning her own real estate business, and began to plan how she could begin her new career. First, she needed to save up enough money to go back to school. She would also have to get a new vehicle. Without one, she would not be able to drive around and show property or for that matter get to church as often as she wanted. She began to save money and set a goal of October to get her new car.

Every morning when she woke, Susan prayed. She prayed on her way to school, on the way back, when she got home, even when she was in the shower. She thanked God for every moment that she was blessed with, moments that she almost lost. Without her faith, she knew that she would have died that day nearly a year ago.

"Hi God, it's Susan again. I'm sure you're sick of hearing this," she would joke, "But thank you." As she prayed, the reason behind the tragedies of that day began to become clearer to her. Maybe what had happened wasn't a lesson for her, but a lesson for the teenaged boy who had crashed into her. He was driving in his mother's car with his friends. Perhaps he was trying to show them how cool he was; how fast he could drive. If she or anyone else had died, his life would have changed forever. Instead of finishing high school, he would be sitting in jail for the rest of his life. What would have happened to his family? Maybe this accident was a wakeup call for him. Or it could have been a wakeup call for someone in her family, showing them that they had a loving family now, but what would happen if they ever lost one of their own? Susan had been close to her brothers and sisters before, but now they were inseparable. Every day they would call each other, just to ask how their day was going. Maybe that was the message that God wanted to give her; that nothing mattered more than family.

I continued to see Susan over the next few months. She was progressing rapidly, and I was hopeful that she would make a full recovery very soon. Her last visit was in August and her father came with her as usual. After looking at her x-rays and examining her we approached the moment I both loved and hated – Susan had improved to the point where she did not need to see me anymore. These moments were always bittersweet as we had forged such a strong bond but at the same time I was so happy to see her improve. Susan laughed with excitement and hugged her dad. As they pulled out of the parking garage for the last time, she logged onto her social media page and posted about her recovery, adding that she had the greatest doctor in the world. She immediately got a flurry of comments. Many of them were from her friends in her choir, whom she constantly stayed in touch with. They asked when she thought she would return to church. "Soon," she promised.

The day before Memorial Day, the anniversary of her accident, arrived. Once again, her father was holding his annual cookout. It was a beautiful day, the kids were excited to swim, and Susan's brothers and sisters were excited to have the fun day they had missed one year earlier due to the accident. So was Susan, but she was scared. She thought about what it would be like to get in the car and buckle up, heading down the same road and sitting at that same intersection waiting for the light to turn green; a green light that served as a metaphor that she was finally allowed to move forward in her life. But then again, what if it didn't? What if the same thing happened, this time ending her life for good? Susan had worked hard to build her life back and she wanted to hold on to it dearly.

As she prepared to head out to the cookout, she remembered what her mother had always told her, and she smiled. "Everything happens for a reason, it is all part of God's plan." As she had done throughout her entire life, Susan moved forward, floating above her struggles with the help of her family, the love of her community, and the power of her faith.

Progress Notes on Susan

Susan continues to live with her sister, spending time adoring her new baby niece. Although she and Larry decided it would be better to be friends, they continue to visit each other and talk every week. She has a new job with a moving company and is working hard on saving money so she can move in to her new home. She feels extremely happy and blessed to be alive.

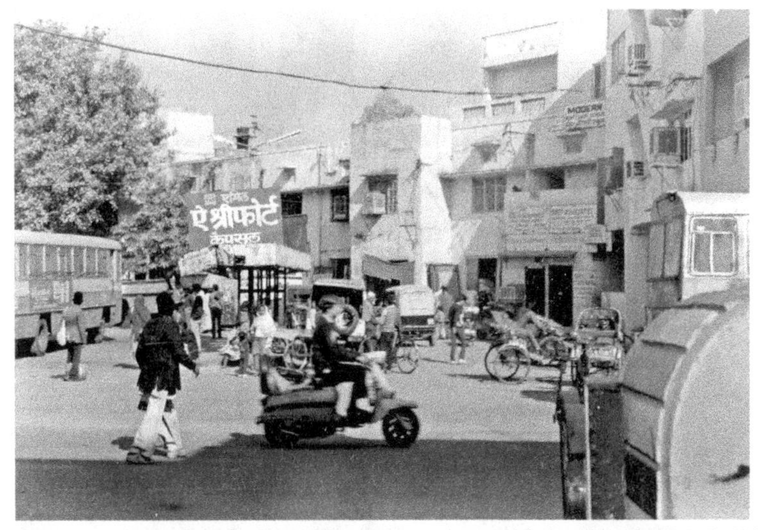

The impoverished neighborhood where my mother and father lived in New Delhi, India. They came to America in search for a better life for their unborn children.

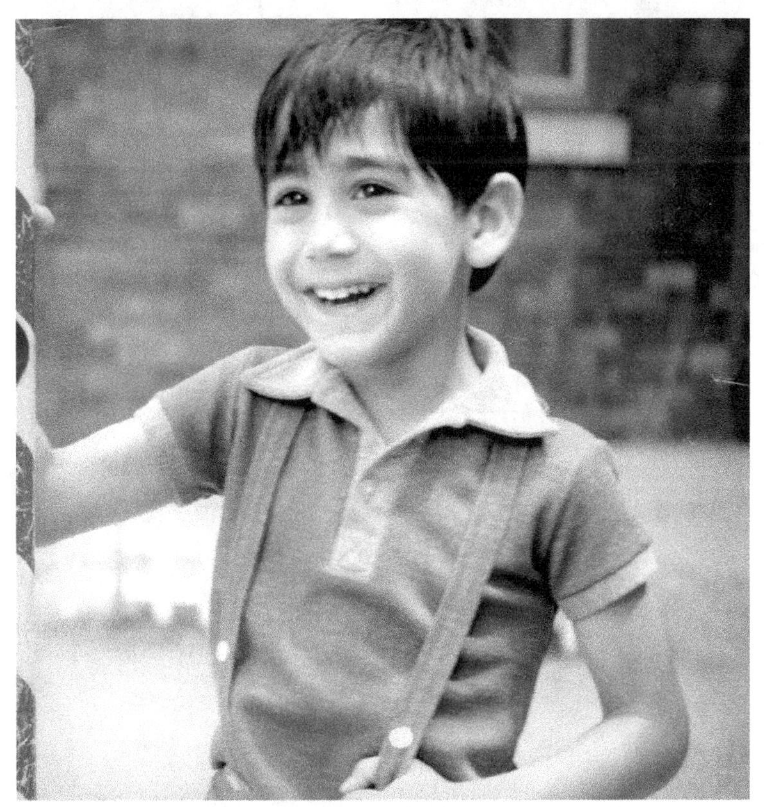

My first day in Kindergarten at Hillsboro Elementary School.

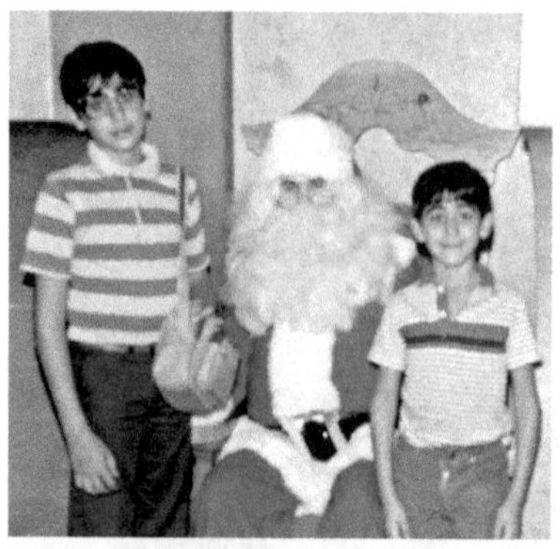

My brother and I spending time with Santa at the annual Coffee County Hospital Christmas Party. I am the little guy on the right.

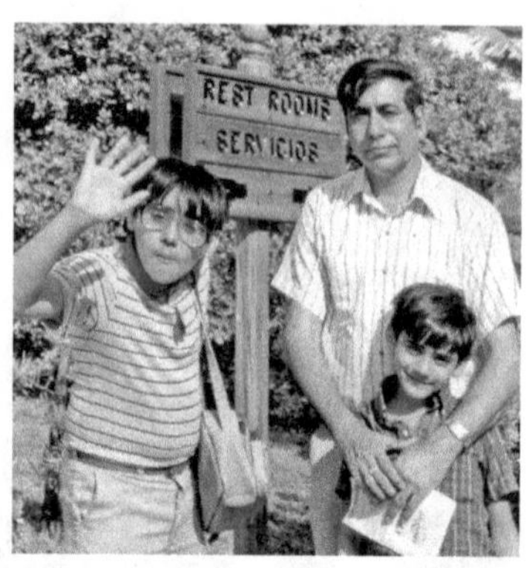

My dad with his arms around me while my brother hams it up for the camera.

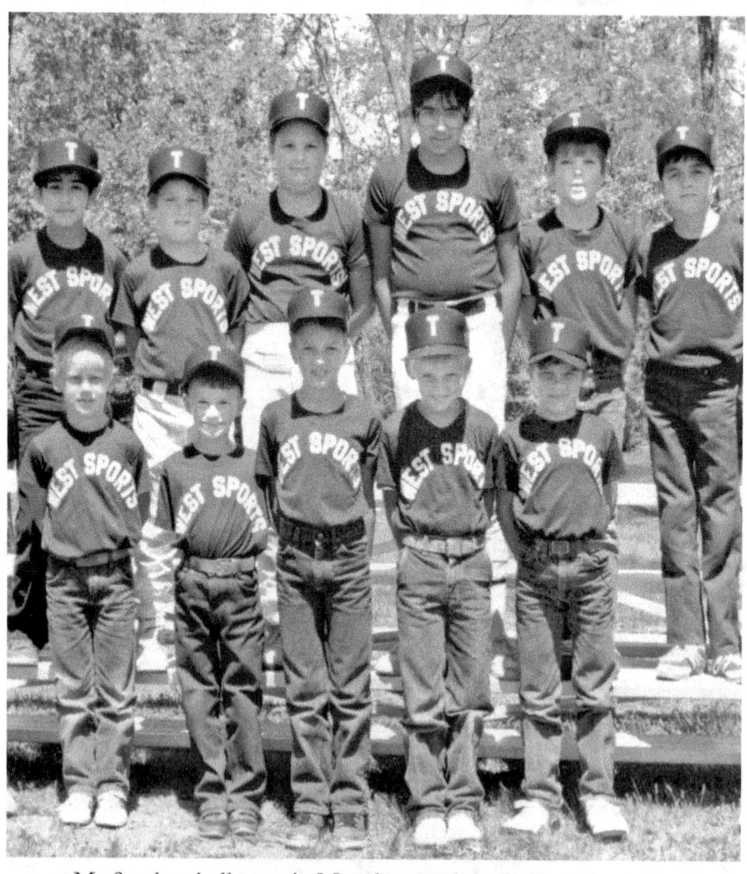

My first baseball team in Manchester where I played first base.
I am on the top left.

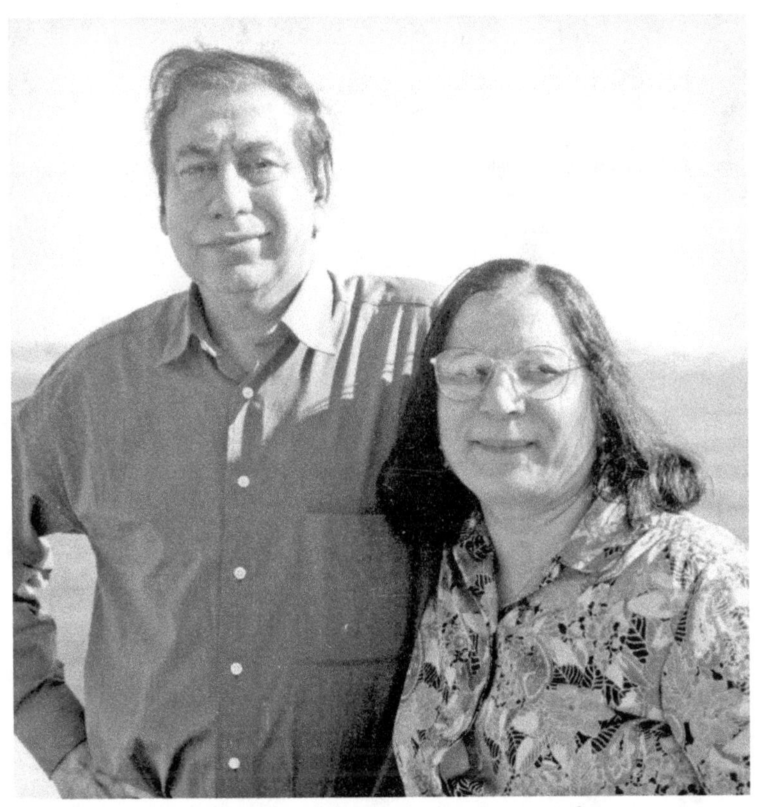

One of my favorite pictures of my parents taken before my father became very sick in 1991.

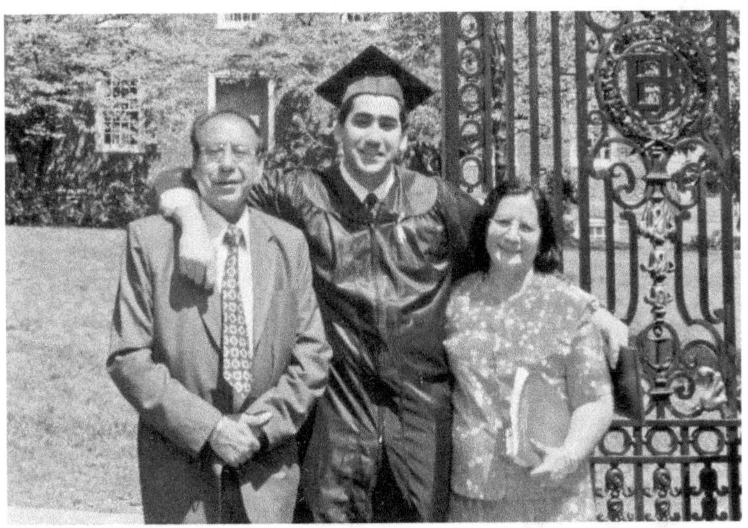

My parents and me at my college graduation.

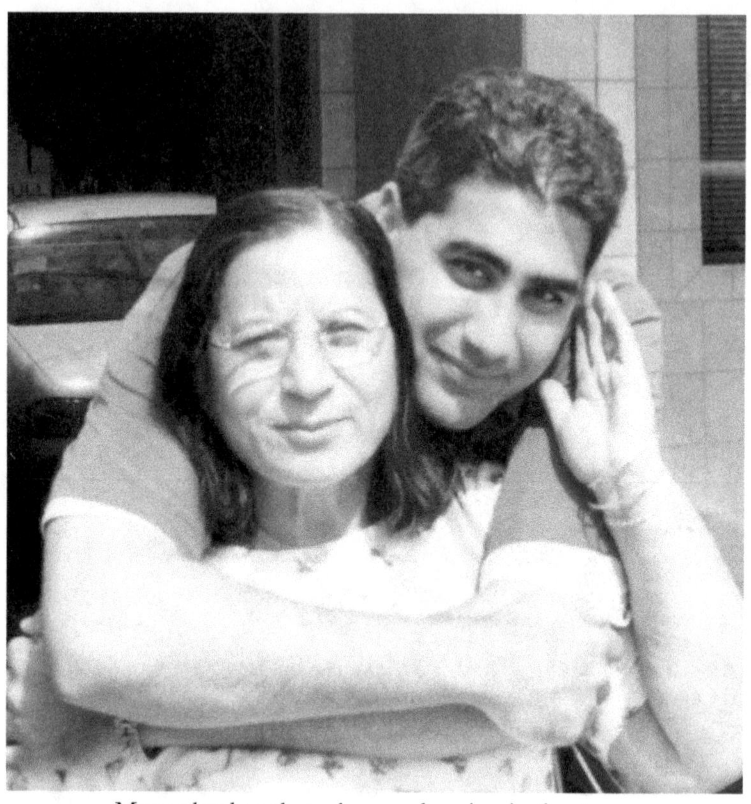

My mother has always been such an inspiration to me
and provides endless love and support.

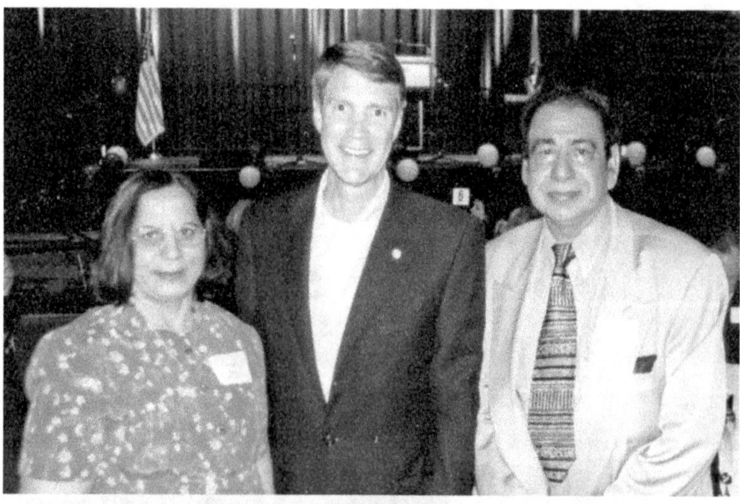

Along with my parents, Senator Frist had a very deep influence on my
growth as a person and as a surgeon. I am grateful for his mentorship.

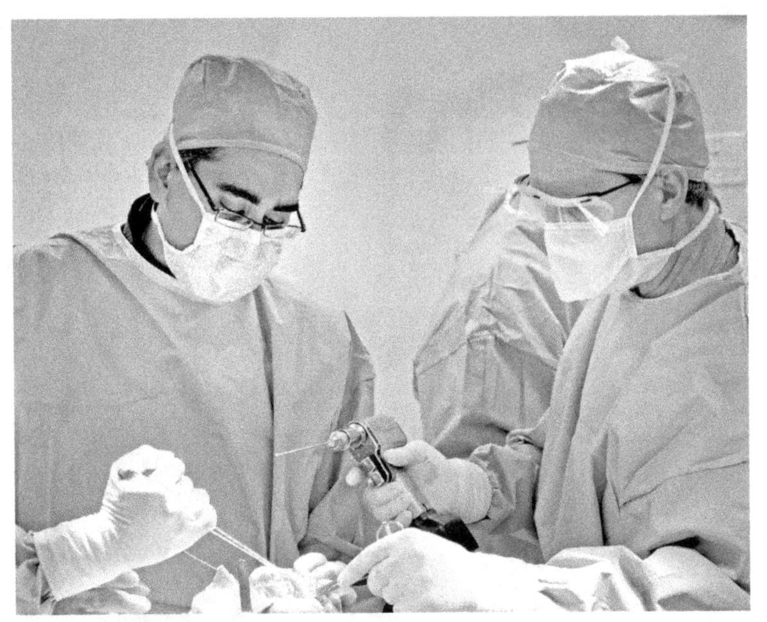

Trauma Fellowship was grueling. Here I am scrubbed with my mentor and friend Dr. Bill Obremskey. He taught me a great deal about management of very sick patients in the operating room.

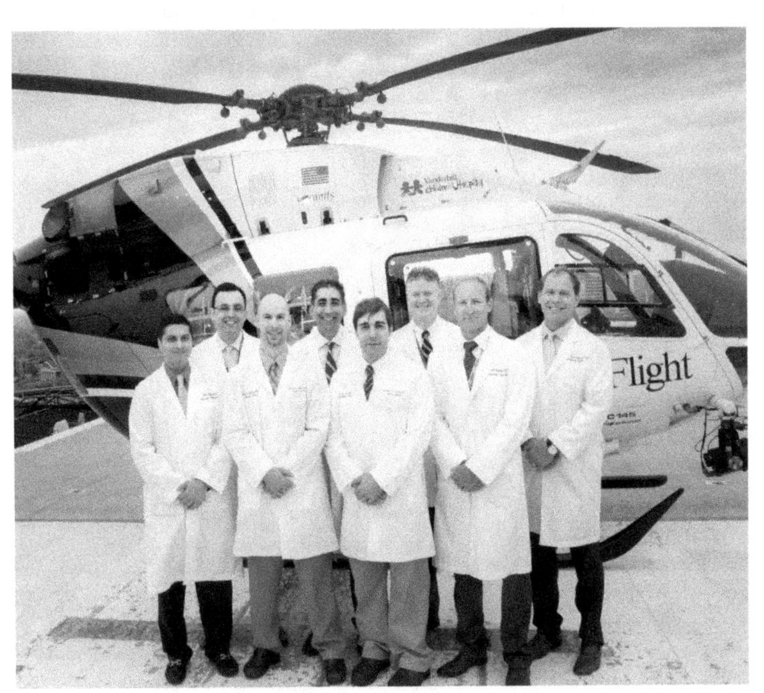

The Orthopedic Trauma Team at Vanderbilt.

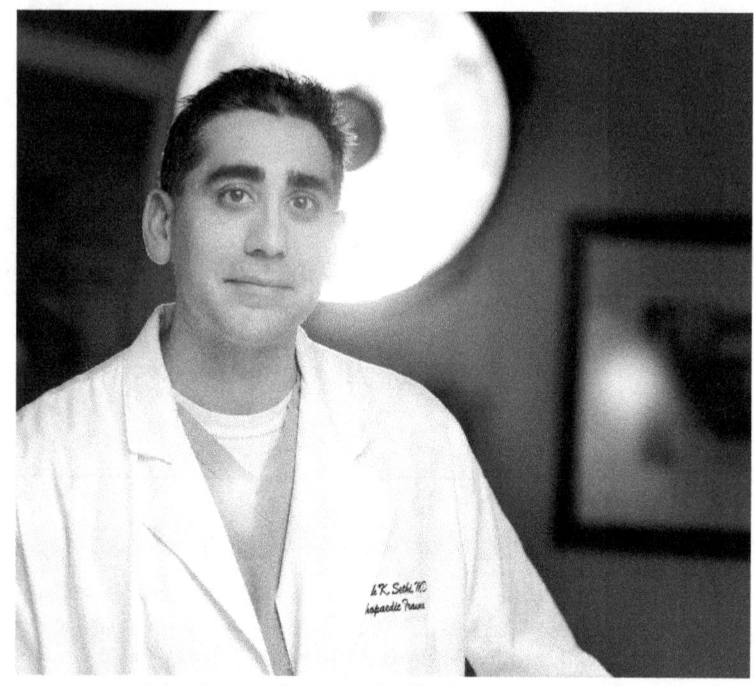

It has been an honor and a blessing to take care of patients as an Orthopedic trauma surgeon at Vanderbilt.

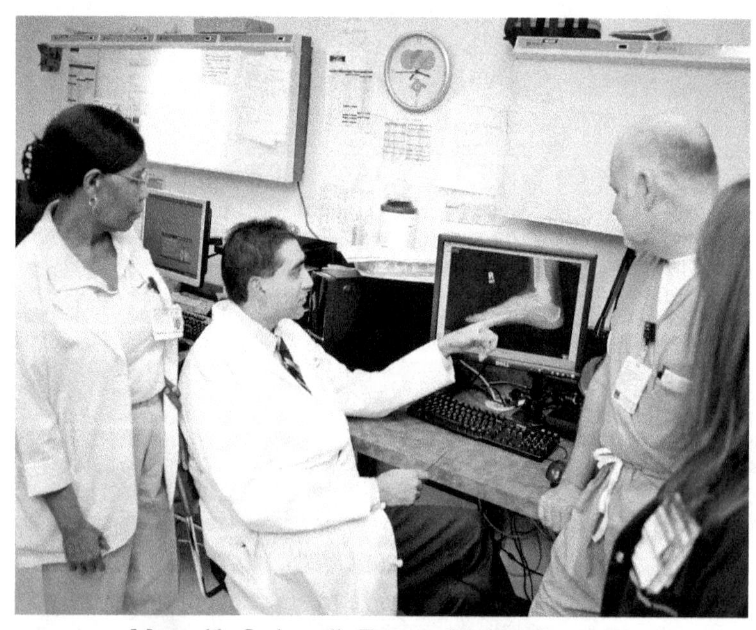

My weekly Orthopedic Trauma Clinic at Vanderbilt where we take care of trauma victims from across Tennessee.

Area Chamber of Commerce
invites you to the
Grand Opening
HEALTHY TENNESSEE

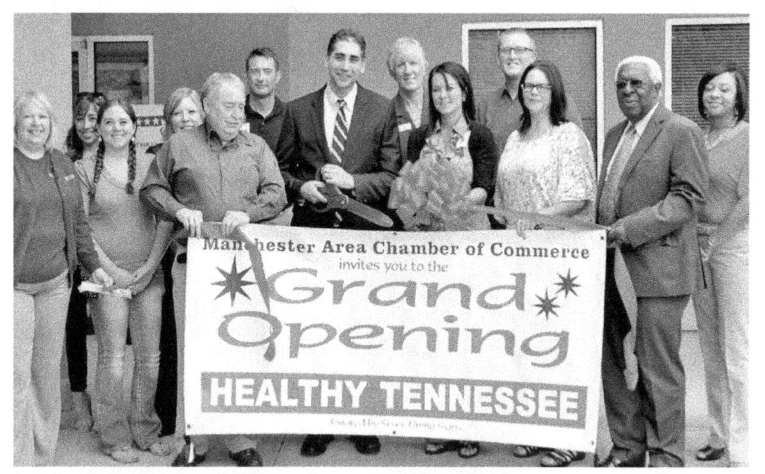

I was so proud to launch our first Healthy Tennessee event in Manchester, where I grew up. Many of the folks in this picture knew me since I was 3 years old. Without them I wouldn't be who I am today.

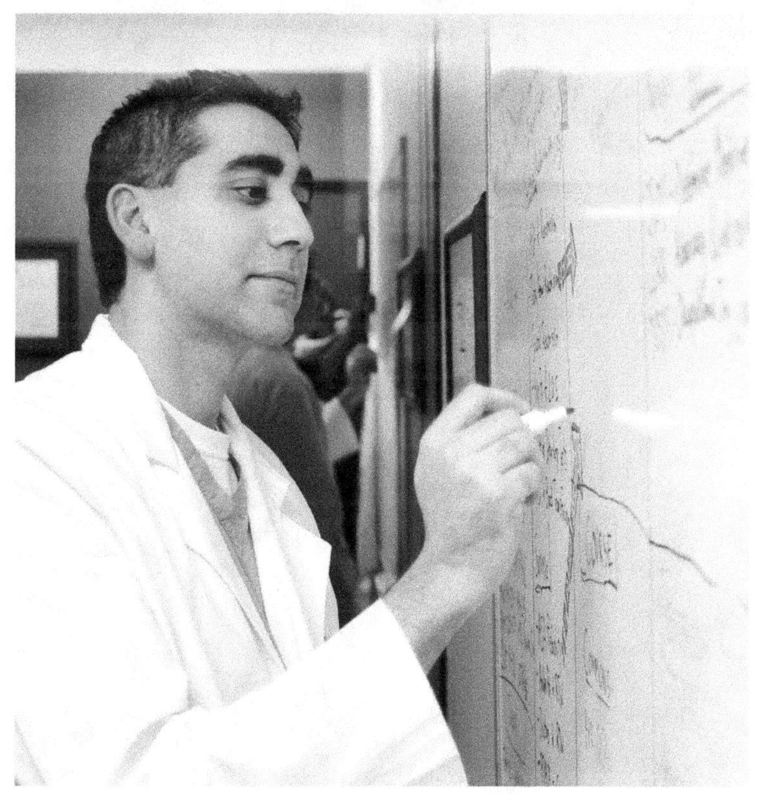

Teaching Vanderbilt undergraduate students and encouraging them to make a difference in the world, its why I chose to become a surgeon.

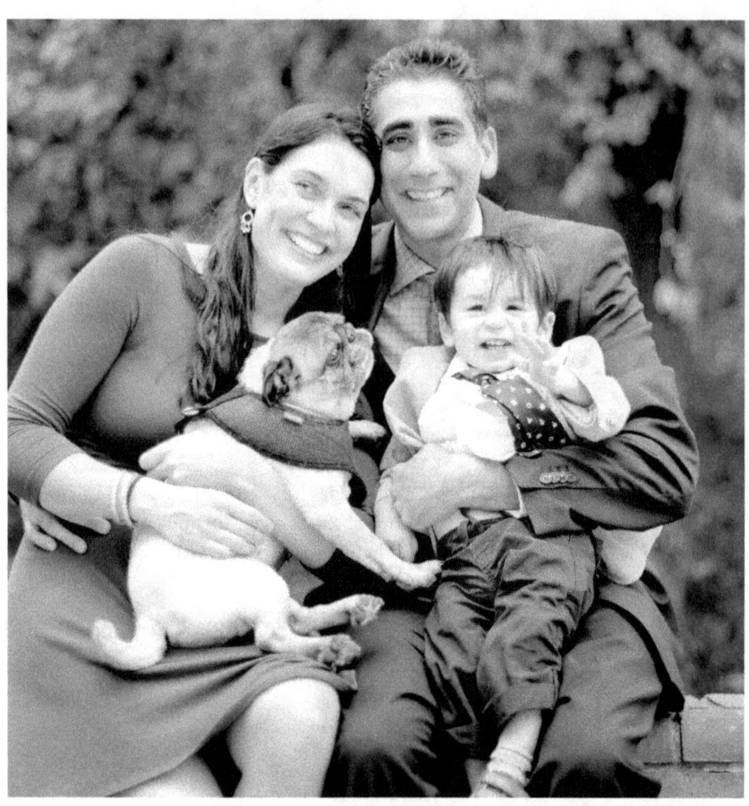

Our little boy JB when he turned one and the love of my life, Maya.

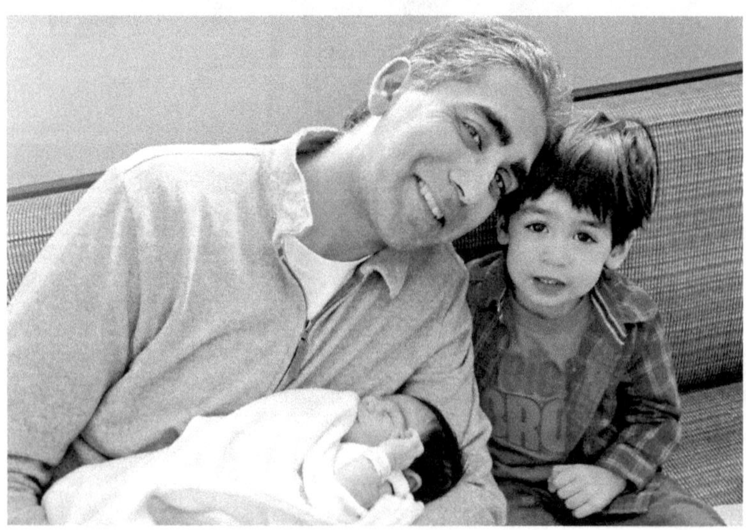

Our growing family; we feel so blessed to
welcome Baby Leela into the world.

Daniel

Fourteen-year old Daniel gazed down the row of pictures that filled the table. They portrayed his uncles, great uncle, grandfather, even his mother, all donned in brown-green camouflage, beaming proudly while they stood in salute. As medicine was to my family's tradition, it was military service to Daniel's.

His uncle, who was sitting in a chair in the living room, noticed him staring at the pictures. "You're in a family of fighters," he added, nodding toward the row of additional photos on the table next to him.

"I guess," said Daniel reluctantly.

His uncle looked at him quizzically. "What's wrong?"

"The school principal saw me doing flips on the playground this morning with Mark and Jackson," Daniel explained. "He said he had never seen anyone with such natural athletic ability. He wants us to put together a gymnastics team and compete with other high school teams. But I've never done gymnastics, why bother now?" Daniel said with a shrug.

"You never give up on anything worth fighting for, son. Whatever you're doing you started off doing for a reason. So you finish it, no matter what," he said.

He knew his uncle was right; they were indeed a family of fighters.

Daniel lived in the 10th ward of the New Orleans projects with his uncle, mother and all of his brothers and sisters. The apartment was a tiny, cramped space, barely enough to fit one person, much less nine. Living in the projects had forced him to grow up much too quickly. Before his grandmother died, he had lived in a comfortable home filled with faith, family, and laughter. Four times a week, without fail, his grandmother would drag him and his eight siblings out of bed and over to the Southern Baptist Church, which was conveniently located next door. Nestled in the pews between his mother and grandmother, he waited anxiously until he could go back home and watch cartoons on television. But sure enough, the next day he was back in the familiar old building that might as well have been his real home. When his grandmother passed away and his mother said they were being forced to leave her home, he wondered if God would follow them where they were going.

Within a few weeks of moving to the projects, Daniel's childlike innocence soon became replaced by a cold, hardened demeanor. You couldn't look soft in the projects, but you couldn't be too hard either or you'd wind up going the wrong way. The only thing he had now was his mother and his siblings. His mother was the rock of the family. He could go to her with any problem, because nine out ten times she would have probably experienced the same thing herself and would know what to do. The only one left to teach him how to be a man was his uncle, since his father had left him long ago. Daniel listened to everything his uncle told him.

Taking his uncle's advice, Daniel and his cousins created a gymnastics team. For the next four years of high school, they won state championships. His uncle's words remained with him through the rest of his life. When he graduated high school, he was given additional wise advice.

"Always stand on your own two feet, and don't ask anyone for anything unless you need it," Daniel's uncle would remind him. "Once you're back on your feet, re-pay it or pay it forward."

Daniel wanted to be able to support himself and make sure that he never ended up in the projects ever again. Following graduation, he attended community college to train to be a nursing assistant. It was while he was working in a nearby nursing home after college that he met Natalie and they dated for a few months. Daniel was content but he knew there was a lot out there and he wanted more in life, just as my mother and father did when they left India in search for a better way of life. Daniel wanted to do something bigger than himself – something with meaning.

On a whim, he decided to move out west and start over. "I don't want to leave New Orleans," Natalie told him simply when he brought it up with her. "Call me if you ever make it back."

Daniel was torn, but the lack of fulfillment he felt with his life in New Orleans was enough to push him to make the move to California. Once there, he worked two jobs, one in retail and one at a small family-owned grocery store. Still, he struggled to make ends meet. He barely had enough to make his monthly rent. Daniel began to feel as if he was just drifting through life once again, directionless with no one to guide him. He thought of his uncle's words, reminding him to never give up. But in the end he accepted defeat, packed up his bags, and headed home.

Upon returning to New Orleans he reunited with Natalie and decided to propose. He hoped settling down would help him feel more stable in life and give him the sense of purpose he desired. After all the struggles he had faced growing up in the projects, he felt he had the strength to do something more with his life. He thought back to the pictures of his military family, and he knew exactly what God had planned for him.

"I'm going to join the military," he told Natalie three months into their marriage.

She narrowed her eyes. "Military means you'll be moving around a lot. I already told you, I'm not interested in leaving New Orleans."

"I know," he said sadly. "But this is what I need to do with my life. I feel it in my gut."

He knew from the start there was a chance he might have to choose between his marriage and the military. When he went into the military office and saw the men and women in uniform bustling around, he felt like he was back home; not the tiny apartment in the projects, but his grandmother's house next to his childhood church.

Within a few months, Daniel had filed all of his paperwork and was officially enlisted. He was assigned to Fort Campbell in Clarksville, Tennessee, just fifty miles north of Nashville. A few weeks later, Natalie filed her own paperwork. Seven months into their marriage, Daniel and Natalie were officially divorced.

With a heavy heart, Daniel set off for Tennessee alone. Fort Campbell was brutal. Daniel wasn't used to people telling him what to do, with him having no choice in the matter. Luckily, he ended up in a unit with great people. The military had a very obvious chain of command, but in his unit, the subordinates and the top officers all worked together. After his first few years, he was assigned to Mannheim, Germany. He loved Fort Campbell, but Mannheim was even better. He met men from other Army units, sometimes even from other countries. By the time he came back to Fort Campbell, he felt like a seasoned soldier. He began working for the 584th Maintenance Company, repairing vehicles. He was starting to feel as if he was finally settling into a comfortable life and began searching for a home near the base. Maybe it was that eight year old inside of him, but when he began searching for the home, he also began searching for a church. He tried out a few different churches, sitting in the pews listening to the pastor's sermon. At most of them, he felt like he was a child again waiting anxiously until he could finally leave. But when he discovered the Concord Baptist Church, it was different. The pastor at the church, Pastor Shaw, was also in the military as were many of the members of the congregation. The first day he went to the church, he met with Pastor Shaw after the sermon. He knew right away that he was the type of person one could talk to about anything and everything.

"I took some wrong turns in life," he admitted to the pastor, thinking of his short-lived marriage. "I need to get my life straight, and that's why I'm here now."

Pastor Shaw nodded. "You have to do it at your own pace," he advised. "But I'm here to help."

Shortly after Daniel found his new home and his new church, his life, like so many others, changed forever on Sept. 11, 2001. Immediately, Daniel received orders to join the Special Forces and the next several years of his life were a whirlwind of special ops training for overseas deployment. Training was especially rough. One day, after jumping over the last rung of a climb ladder in a conditioning course, he lost his balance and fell down hard on his knee. The pain was overwhelming but in the military, you learn quickly that pain is a state of mind, and that you push through it no matter what. So he jumped back up and masked the pain that began throbbing uncontrollably throughout his leg. It was an injury that would later come back to haunt him.

While continuing to train for overseas deployment he met a group that he quickly considered his brothers and sisters. It was a motorcycle club and his chief officer in the military, Rick, was the president of the group. The clubhouse, which was a large, quaint home, was situated on a cozy street off the highway. It was Rick's living quarters but was also used as an informal gathering place for the club. When he had first heard that most of his unit was in this motorcycle club, Daniel was a little concerned. Since he had re-joined the church, he no longer drank or smoked and he feared he would be tempted to do both with a bunch of bikers. But Daniel soon learned there was more to the club then just riding and partying. The club was in fact, a family of brothers and sisters in arms who all shared the same passion for riding. Tyler and Jim became two of his closest friends in the group. Sadie, one of the few females in the group, behaved like an older sister in the way she protectively looked over him.

Daniel had ridden motorcycles before, so he knew how to ride and once he joined the club he bought his own. Speeding down the highway freed his mind and gave him a sense of clarity in a way that nothing else had been able to do. Every weekend, the club would ride from Clarksville to Nashville, turn around and ride back. The sense of camaraderie he felt during those rides was amazing. Ten years earlier, Daniel feared he would drift aimlessly through life, sad and alone. Now, there were three things that Daniel couldn't imagine his life without; his motorcycle club, the military, and his church.

After further training, the time for Daniel and his unit to be sent overseas was approaching. A few months before their departure, Daniel was carrying a large, bulky safe up the stairs when he felt his leg suddenly give out. He fell to the floor along with the safe with a large thud.

"What happened?" Rick asked, rushing to him.

"I don't know," Daniel responded, wincing in pain. "My leg just gave out. I'll be fine though," he responded, moving to get himself back up.

"I don't think so," Rick said sternly. "You're going to the hospital."

Daniel didn't want to go. He feared if the doctors found something wrong, he would not be allowed to deploy.

Listening to Rick's advice, he went and when the doctor pulled up his x-ray and began explaining to Daniel what had happened, his worst fears were confirmed.

"Both your left knee and femur are fractured."

"How did that happen?" Daniel asked incredulously.

"You've lost a lot of cartilage in your knee cap, which makes me think this fracture must have happened a long time ago. Can you think of anytime when you might have fallen hard on your knee?"

Daniel flashed back to the time when he fell off the ladder climb. He knew that must have been it. The doctor informed him that he would need surgery to fix his leg. His heart sank. That meant that all of his brothers and sisters would deploy, doing their part to serve their country, while he remained disabled back home.

The next year was full of uncertainty. Following his surgery, Daniel went to rehab every day, working on regaining the full strength and use of his leg. The pain that shot through his leg every time he exercised was excruciating, but he pretended it was nothing. He was informed by his officers that due to his injury, there was a good chance that he would be discharged. He knew he couldn't let that happen, so he endured the pain like he had been taught to do for all these years.

Following a year of intense rehab, Daniel was allowed to join his unit in the Middle East. He was placed on the P2 profile, which meant that he still wasn't allowed to run or go into combat. The bone that was used to fix his knee was cadaver bone, which could easily become dislodged in combat. Every day was a struggle for Daniel, but he still worked through the pain. At night when he laid in bed, his leg would eventually become numb after hours of throbbing with pain. Still, being there with his brothers meant more to him than anything.

When Daniel returned to Clarksville, Tennessee from overseas, he met Christina, who would soon become his second wife. Soon after they married, she gave birth to twin boys. As he held them in his arms for the first time, he realized they were the greatest gift that had ever been bestowed to him. It wasn't long though, until the strain of being a military wife began to wane on Christina. A year into their marriage, Daniel was deployed for another year, and she was left behind at home alone with the boys. As with his first wife, Christina began to resent his military career. She asked him to quit the military.

"I can't leave," he pleaded with her when he returned from his deployment. "You don't understand. The military means everything to me."

"More than your family?" she asked.

Daniel didn't know what to do. Now, he had others to think about; his wife and his two kids. But the military had given him his sense of purpose in life, and they were also his family. How could he just leave them?

Daniel needed to think, so he geared up his bike and sped off down the highway to help clear his head. It was Memorial Day weekend, so the streets were packed. There was bumper to bumper traffic. As he approached the intersection of Preachers Mill Road and Highway 101, he glanced at a Dodge Ram truck that was standing at a stop sign. Daniel continued across the intersection. Suddenly and without warning, the truck pulled into the middle of the road in front of Daniel. His motorcycle smashed into the truck, sending Daniel over the hood and plummeting to the hard highway surface.

He breathed heavily as he lay on his back, staring up at the clouds. Dark red blood began to ooze across his uniform, an all too familiar sight from his tours in the Middle East that made his stomach queasy. The pain was unnerving and was greater than anything he had ever faced in combat. As a soldier, his first instinct was to immediately stand up and get off the road, but the moment he tried to move, a sharp pain ran through his leg. He looked down and was horrified. The bottom of his shoe was twisted up into his thigh.

The streets became filled with the distant wail of sirens and strangely, the heavy roar of motorcycles. Daniel began shaking while the world spun around him. When he opened his eyes, he was shocked to see his friends from the Army, Tyler and Jim, kneeling next to him. He opened his mouth to speak but he couldn't. Everything went black.

The next sound Daniel heard was the roar of a helicopter. He had a quick flash back and for a second thought he was back in the Middle East, and immediately thought he must have been hurt in combat. He looked around in a daze. His leg throbbed with unbearable pain. He felt a sharp prick to his arm, and he fell back out of consciousness.

By the time Daniel arrived at Vanderbilt Hospital, I was up to date on his status. He was initially taken to the military hospital where after seeing the severity of the damage the doctors felt they had no choice but to amputate his leg in order to save his life. Luckily, one of the other doctors intervened and told them to take him to Vanderbilt. Upon arriving at our hospital, he was taken immediately to the operating room where I examined his wounds. He had a large open wound on his lower leg, and both his knee and tibia were badly fractured. The pressure was cutting off blood supply to his leg, a condition called compartment syndrome. If this continued to happen, the muscles and nerves would die off and we would have to cut off his leg. We operated and stabilized his leg, releasing all of the pressure on the muscles so that blood could flow freely once more.

As we finished the surgery and I went downstairs to the waiting area to talk with his family I thought about the long journey that Daniel would face in saving his leg and what I would tell his family. These were always such hard conversations but very important as it was Daniel's family that would play a critical role in his recovery.

When Daniel woke the next morning, the first thing he noticed was a man in a military uniform standing in the far corner of the room. He was wide-eyed and his face was pale.

"Who are you?" Daniel murmured.

"I'm Quincy," he said softly. "I'm the man who hit you."

Daniel had a thousand questions, but he was overcome with a sense of dizziness and the room became black. For the next few days Daniel continued to fall in and out of consciousness as his body struggled to recover. Every day I checked on him to see how he was progressing. He still needed another surgery to cover his wounds, but we had to wait until he was stabilized.

Daniel's mother and his sisters stayed with him every day he was in the hospital. There was always someone from his motorcycle club there as well. Over time, however, the panic from nearly losing her son was too much for Daniel's mother to bear, and she began to have severe asthma attacks. She was hospitalized a few floors away from Daniel. His sisters went from room to room, trying to care for them both. Without fail, Quincy was a presence in the corner of the room.

Four days after his initial surgery, I took Daniel back to the operating room where we examined his leg and took skin from his thigh to cover the large incisions we had made. Following surgery we talked and I told Daniel what we had done. He was very worried about losing his leg and I assured him that we would do everything to save it. I also told him that he would need further surgery down the road to replace all of the bone he lost during the accident. As he started to weep, I looked him in the eye and told him to hold onto his faith and things would work out.

When I left the room, Daniel turned his attention to Quincy who as usual was standing in the corner. For the first time since he was in the hospital, Daniel had the strength to talk to him.

"Which unit are you in?" Daniel asked, nodding toward his uniform.

"Unit 18," he replied, walking slowly up toward Daniel. "I just want to say how sorry I am." His voice quivered slightly. "I shouldn't have gone into that intersection, I should have waited."

Daniel was silent. "I understand," he said finally.

"You don't have to say that," Quincy began.

But Daniel cut him off, "The Lord chose me to go through this in life. I'm not going to make it hard on somebody else, especially not you. You and I are the same brothers in arms."

Quincy gave him a faint smile of appreciation.

Daniel continued to recover in the hospital for a few more days before he was discharged. He would remain in a wheelchair for at least the next four months. After the accident, things became more intense between him and his wife. She hoped that now that he was injured, he'd consent to leave the military.

"I didn't leave the first time I hurt my leg, and I'm not leaving this time," he told her when he arrived home. After a few days at home, he moved to his sister's house where both she and his mom could take care of him while Christina took care of the kids. While there, Pastor Shaw began visiting him twice a week.

"Stay strong," he assured him. "Most importantly, keep your faith. It will get you through all the trials and tribulations ahead of you."

"I know," Daniel answered. "I never questioned, and I never will."

He began going to rehab three times a week. The exercises were painful to do while sitting in his wheelchair, so they recommended he do pool therapy. As soon as he got in the water and began moving around, he began to feel better. I can do this, he thought, I can get better.

Daniel was becoming restless. He not only wanted to go back to work, but he wanted to get back on his bike. Luckily, he was still able to go to church every week. The first Sunday he returned, his sister wheeled him up to the front and put him on the display for everyone to see. The older ladies in the front pews jumped up and began smothering him with kisses. It was nice to see how much they missed him, but even nicer to sit in the pews and hear Pastor Shaw speak and be a part of the congregation. After church, his sisters from the club, Sadie and Tammy, went over to him and told him they were taking him out for the day.

"But where can I go?" Daniel asked.

"Anywhere you want! You're not just going to sit around the house all day." The girls taking him out for the day became a regular thing that he looked forward to.

Most of the time, they took him to see the motorcycle races. As he watched the bikes zoom by, he felt a rush of adrenaline. He couldn't wait to get back on his bike.

"You're crazy," his sister Charlotte said when he told her he was planning to ride again. "You can't go back on that bike! Not after this!"

"You remember what Uncle Kevin would say? We don't give up on things. If we set out to do it for a reason, then it's worth fighting for."

"But riding?" she questioned.

"It's not just the riding. The camaraderie I have with the guys makes my life better. I didn't have any friends before this. You know that. I kept to myself and just went to work and came home and repeated that cycle every day. That's not living. That's just being. And I don't want that."

After a few months of therapy, Daniel came back to Vanderbilt for his last surgery. We were able to transplant bone from his femur and insert it into his tibia where the defect was. The surgery was a success and Daniel was on his way to recovery. He had come very far quickly because of his strong faith and the love from his family and biking community.

Daniel was ecstatic. After a few more weeks doing pool therapy, the military requested that he return to the rehab facility in Clarksville so they could begin monitoring his progress. After a few more weeks of therapy, he was finally able to walk on crutches.

"Now I can go back to work," he told his commanding officer, Sergeant Jefferson.

"We think the wheelchair will be better," he responded. "Come in tomorrow, we'll find you a desk job where you can stay for a few months."

Daniel didn't want to regress and go back to the wheelchair, but he'd take whatever he could get. He just wanted to go back to work. The next morning he got dressed in his uniform and his sister took him to the base. When Daniel got to the offices, he realized how difficult this was truly going to be. The floor was concrete, which made wheeling around more difficult. Even worse, he had to keep his leg straightened out for the next few months in order for it to heal. With his leg propped up on the seat beside him, Daniel ended up using two desk spaces instead of one. It seemed to him that he was a bigger hindrance there than he was at home. For the first time, he began to get nervous. If he didn't recover soon, the Army could transfer him into the wounded warrior program. The program was meant to help soldiers transition into civilian life or go back to work in the military depending on the severity of their injuries, but Daniel knew it was mostly the former. In Christina's eyes, the program was a blessing, but for Daniel it was a death sentence.

"I don't want to leave the military," Daniel told her after his first day on his new desk job. "I'm going back, I have to."

The thought of him returning to the military was overwhelming to her. "Maybe you shouldn't move back home after you recover," she said sadly. "Maybe it's time for us to move on."

Daniel was heart-broken. This was his second marriage broken up because of his desire to stay in the military. The military was his purpose; what would he do instead? The only other thing he felt as passionate about was riding, but he might end up even losing that if he didn't get better. He knew he should be thankful that he made it out of that accident alive, but if he wasn't able to do the things he loved, what was the point?

Daniel remained at his sister's house. He continued to go to work in the military office for the next few months. He also came back to my clinic a few times, where I checked on his progress.

"Do I look any better?" he asked hopefully every time I came back into the room after examining his x-ray. Over time Daniel's leg healed but he was not completely back to where he was physically before the accident. He was eager to walk without a limp and to continue his active military career. It was a hard conversation to have, but I told him that he may never be able to walk without a limp given the extensive trauma he had faced; I was glad we had saved his leg.

But Daniel was distraught. "I can't be in the military with a cane!"

He began to panic. During the next few weeks, he put all his effort into trying to get off the crutches. He felt the pressure to get better as quickly as possible, before the Army would give up on him. But he knew he couldn't push himself too hard or he would end up hurting himself further. It was a delicate balance. Finally, after hours of intense rehab, Daniel was able to begin walking with a cane. He began to feel optimistic again. That's why, when he was called into his commanding officer's office one day during work, he expected good news.

"I'm afraid I have bad news," Sergeant Jefferson began. "We've been talking to your therapist, and she said there's a good chance that your leg is going to end up being a P3, maybe even a P4."

Daniel shook his head. A P3 would mean that he wouldn't be

able to run and grab his weapon, all the things they needed him to do. A P4 would mean that they would have to discharge him. His other leg was already a P2, which means he was limited in what he could do. "No, I'll get better."

His commanding officer looked regretful. "I'm sorry. There are no more options now. We have to move you to the wounded warrior program."

Daniel felt as if he had just been stabbed in the back. After more than a decade of service, they were going to discharge him. "Yes, sir," he responded bitterly.

When Daniel returned to therapy the next day, he felt defeated. He continued his exercises with his cane. At this point he knew his military career was over. Now, he just had to try to get off the cane so he could still have some semblance of a normal life. But as he walked from one side of the room to the other, the throbbing in his leg would be so bad that he'd have to stop and sit down.

"You should try not putting weight on the cane. You should only use it for stability," his therapist reminded him.

"I know, but I can't," he said sadly. "I just can't do it."

After another month, it became apparent that Daniel was going to progress no further. He was discharged from therapy, and with that, discharged from the Army. Daniel felt like he had lost everything. He would have to use his cane for the rest of his life. That afternoon, he visited Rick in his garage, where he fixed motorcycles as a side job. "That's tough," Rick said when he heard the news. "Can you still ride?"

"I don't know," Daniel said. The truth was, he was afraid to try. He already lost his wife and his career. He couldn't lose riding too.

"I don't know how you're dealing with all of this, to be honest," Rick admitted.

"Faith," he answered. "I feel like I'm living in a world where someone is constantly trying to kill me. Without my faith, I wouldn't be standing here today."

Rick nodded, contemplating Daniel's words as he wiped off the front of the bike he had just repaired. "I'm glad you're here. I have something for you."

Rick went to the back of his garage to a bike in the corner, which was covered with a sheet. He removed the sheet. Underneath was Daniel's old bike, bright and shiny.

Daniel looked incredulous. "You fixed it?"

"Yeah, it wasn't too badly damaged. Since it just slid under the truck, it needed only minor repairs. I hope it works though, I don't really have any experience fixing hogs."

"I do," Daniel said, "I dabbled with mine a bit." He walked up to the bike "This looks great, Rick, thank you," he exclaimed. "You know, you could really expand your business if you started fixing hogs. There are a lot of guys who ride these as well."

Rick smiled knowingly. "You're right. It's about time we do something about this." He held out his hand. "Partners?"

Daniel smiled back at him. Then, he clasped his hand and shook it firmly. His future suddenly became clear to him. That night, he began researching schools where he could train to be a motorcycle mechanic. He found one in Florida that would be relatively quick and inexpensive. Now, all he needed to do was to get there and find a place to stay for a few months while he trained. He was overcome by a familiar feeling. It was the same feeling he felt when he realized that he wanted to join the military. He finally had a sense of purpose again. The one problem was figuring out how he would get to Florida. All he had was his motorcycle; his wife had taken the car when she left. Riding to Florida would have been a piece of cake before. If he was going to drive down there, he had to finally get on his bike.

The next morning, Daniel headed over to the club house. The crew was planning on riding to Nashville that day. In the driveway sat his bike that Rick had fixed. Most of the crew was already lined up ready to drive off. When they saw Daniel, they cheered.

"You're riding with us today?" Sadie asked. "Are you sure?"

Daniel nodded as he climbed onto his bike. He thought of his uncle's words. He extended his leg forward and rested it comfortably on the peg. He said a quick prayer before gearing up his bike. The familiar rumbling sound felt like music to his ears. Slowly, he lifted his other leg and moved forward, lining up next to the rest of the crew.

"Ready to ride?" Rick asked.

Daniel nodded. "I am," he said confidently. He geared up his bike one more time. Together once again, they sped off into the horizon.

Progress Notes on Daniel

Daniel lives in Clarksville and continues to ride with his friends in the motorcycle club several times a week. He continues to remain strong in his faith and still hopes to start his own motorcycle repair shop in the coming years.

Evan

"I don't think you should go running today," Sarah said as she sat at their kitchen table, looking at Evan nervously as he tied his shoes.

"You know I have to," Evan responded.

"I have a bad feeling," she added, her forehead wrinkled with worry.

"Trust me; nothing bad is going to happen. What are the chances of that? I've run up and down these streets plenty of times."

She looked at him doubtfully. Evan walked over and planted a kiss on Sarah's forehead. "I'm not going right now anyway. Mom is picking me up and we are going into town for my physical."

One month after high school, Evan had moved in with his high school sweetheart, Sarah. The first thing Evan did after graduating was go to the military office in town. He had spent his high school years training and toning his body so he could join the Army. The first day he did a weigh in, they told him that he looked good, but needed to shed two more inches off his gut. For the next two months, all Evan did was train to do just that. When he had returned to the military office, they told him he was ready.

"Go ahead and finish up the rest of the enlistment process, just make sure you don't do anything to regain the weight in the meantime," the officer had cautioned.

For the last two weeks, he was running five miles a day to stay in shape. Today, he was getting an updated physical, one of the last things to do before he could officially enlist. After that, he would meet his friend Martin at Montgomery Bell State Park so they could go swimming.

Evan's mom pulled up to his house, and the two headed to town. He passed his physical with flying colors and when the doctor weighed him, Evan breathed a sigh of relief as he realized he hadn't gained any weight from his last weigh in. Within an hour, his appointment was over and he felt like he was on top of the world. Now, all he had to do was have the military call him to tell him that they had processed all of his paperwork and could move forward with his application.

"You look happy," his mom said as they got into the car.

"I am," he beamed back at her. "Actually, you know what? I think I'll jog to Montgomery Bell. It's about five miles and I haven't gone for my run today."

"Are you sure?"

"Yeah, it will be good. I'll call you to come get me if I get tired."

"All right," she said hesitantly. "But be careful on the road."

"I will," Evan promised, before he turned and ran off. Finishing that physical had made Evan realize how far he had truly come. He was no longer the chubby kid the kids teased in middle school. More than that, he knew exactly what he wanted to do in life and where he was headed. He turned at the intersection and began to jog down the long road to the state park, a road lined on both sides by dense woods. As he continued running at a fast pace he thought of Jake looking down at him from heaven. Evan couldn't help but beam with pride.

Suddenly, an immense pain shot across Evan's leg, quickly spreading across his entire body. He was thrown into the air. Within seconds, he landed with a large thud in the ditch. Everything went black.

"Just 10 more to go Evan, then you're done!"

Evan gazed up at Jake's face. His forehead dripping with sweat, Evan let out a deep growl before lifting the weights high above his chest.

"31! Keep going Evan!"

"I can't do it!" Evan yelled.

"Yes you can, I believe in you."

Evan lifted the weights again, using every ounce of strength in his body. He flashed back to an image of his reflection in the mirror one year earlier; his round face and oversized shirt that clung tightly to his body would remain forever ingrained in his mind. In the sixth grade at the time, nothing mattered more to Evan than losing weight and impressing the other boys and girls in his class. Although he was only a little bit chubby, he was tired of being picked on for his weight. Soon after his parents had divorced, his mother began dating a man named Frank. When Frank noticed Evan's insecurities, he connected him with a local trainer he knew named Jake who offered to help get Evan into shape.

Over the next year, Evan trained with Jake every day at the gym. Over time, he became like the older brother Evan had always wanted but never had. Although his mother had given birth to another boy after him, he died soon after birth. With five younger sisters, Evan knew more about dolls and make-up than any boy should. He and his oldest sister, Sherry, were always wrestling as if they were brothers. Still, Evan longed for an older brother to guide him through life. After his parents had divorced, Evan had become very close to his step-mother, Jeanie. His birth mother could never understand his problems and he was never very close to his father. The majority of their conversations began with "yes sir," and the rest with "no, sir." Evan knew his father must love him, but he never showed it. That was why it meant so much to Evan when Jake offered to take him under his wing.

After a year of hard work, Evan went from being the last kid picked in gym class to the first one across the finish line at the end of every race. The girls in his class started noticing him for the first time, which made him feel like the most popular boy in Creek Wood, Tennessee. That wasn't really saying much; the entirety of Creek Wood could fill the pews in a mid-sized church.

By the time Evan entered the eighth grade, he was a completely different person. He felt like he was on top of the world. He wasn't particularly religious and his mother left the choice of going to church up to him, but he still thanked God almost every night for bringing Jake into his life. Things changed suddenly when his mother came into his room one night. She said to Evan, "I have some terrible news about Jake." Evan's heart sank into his stomach.

"What's wrong?" Evan said, his voice quivering.

"Frank just talked to Jake on the phone. The doctors found a tumor in his brain. They said he only has a few months to live."

Evan's world was turned upside down with the news. The next few months were the worst of his life. Every day when he went to see Jake in the hospital, he saw his friend become smaller and weaker. The muscular, energetic Jake that he knew was replaced by a frail, dying young man. Evan couldn't take it. He still mourned the one brother that he lost before he even got a chance to know him. Losing Jake was much worse.

By the time Evan graduated from middle school, Jake had passed away. Evan was numb with pain. "Why don't you go for a run, Evan? Going for runs always made you happy," his step-mother would say to try to get him out of bed.

Evan would merely roll over and turn his back to her, tears forming in his eyes. It was impossible for Evan to go for a run, or to the gym. Jake had taught him everything that he had known about training. Now, he was gone.

By the time he was a freshman in high school; Evan had changed again and appeared to be a completely different person. He befriended a circle of misfits, other outsiders like himself who did whatever they wanted whenever they wanted. It was with them that he had his first sip of beer, followed by a shot of whiskey and a cigarette. Before long, Evan was skipping school to get drunk and to smoke with his friends. He was bitter and angry with life, picking fights with most of the people he met. Now in a deep depression, he ate incessantly. His tall, muscular build soon returned to its weaker, chubbier self.

After a year of avoiding training, Evan weighed close to four-hundred pounds. He went from the fastest to the fattest kid in in his class. By the time he entered high school, his weight made him stick out like a sore thumb. In fact, the only person that even came close to his size was Martin, a new boy who had just moved to Creek Wood. Although Martin didn't fit in with the popular kids, there was one pretty girl that Evan would always see him with. One day, when he saw Martin in the hallway, hugging the pretty brunette before she left for class, he decided to approach him, a sneer on his face.

"Who are you?" He asked.

"My name is Martin, I just moved here."

"Who was that girl you were just hugging? Is that your girlfriend? There's no way that's your girlfriend."

Martin gave him an icy glare. "That was my sister."

Evan scoffed. "I knew it," he said with a smirk before walking away.

For some reason, Evan couldn't help but tease Martin. Maybe it was because it helped him forget about all the people who were constantly teasing him. Even outside of school, Martin couldn't escape Evan's bullying. For the next year of his life, Evan spent most of his time smoking in the parking lots, vandalizing town buildings, and drinking every night of the weekend. Evan knew what he was doing was wrong, but he didn't care. The only person who gave him a twinge of guilt was his mother.

"Evan, please talk to me," she would beg him when he came home late at night, smelling the whiskey on his breath. He would shrug her off and head to his room. "Think of what Jake would say," she whispered one day as he walked up the stairs.

Evan paused on the steps. After a few seconds, he continued up to his room. When he got there, he turned on his light and looked at himself in the mirror. He sighed. What would Jake have said? He worked so hard to help Evan get in shape, to help him feel good about himself. Now, Evan was in even worse shape, drinking, smoking, and failing his classes. What had happened to his dreams of traveling the world, of going to college? Evan wished there was someone in his life that could help him. He began to wonder how many other people there were in the world like him, mourning the loss of a friend with no one to turn to. Evan clenched his fists and punched the mirror as hard as he could watching it shatter.

The next day, when Evan arrived to school, a poster hanging on the wall next to the office caught his eye. He walked up to it. A man in uniform with his hand up in salute peered off into the horizon. Behind him was the ocean and above it, written across the blue sky, was the word "Navy." Suddenly, in that one moment, everything became clear to him. The Navy. He was going to join the Navy.

The majority of Evan's family had served in the military and he saw it as his best shot at getting out of his small town and travel the world. Evan wanted to go places: Japan, Europe, anywhere other than the twenty-mile radius where he had spent the entirety of his life. Now, he began to see a new vision for his life as a member of the Navy. He looked down at himself and after seeing his protruding belly, he nearly laughed. There was no way he could join the Navy in this kind of shape. If he was truly going to join the Navy after high school, he had to commit now. He had to go back to the Evan he was when Jake was alive. Evan clenched his fists, determined.

When Evan left school that day, he ignored his friends in the parking lot who were beckoning him to join them for a smoke.

Instead, he went straight to his car and following a short drive, he was back in front of that familiar building where he had trained with Jake. He sat in the car for a few minutes, listening to the silent hum of the engine. Then, he turned off his car and walked inside.

"I'd like a year-long membership please," he said to the receptionist, slapping his ID and credit card onto the counter in front of her.

Within a short time, Evan was once again headed in the right direction, both mentally and physically. Every day after school, he would go to the gym and lift weights. During lunchtime at school, he would run around the track. It wasn't easy at first. He nearly collapsed after his first lap. He thought back to middle school, when he could literally run circles around the other students while they gasped for air. It hurt, but he was determined and he kept on running. More than anything, Evan worked on his leg muscles. He knew having strong and sturdy legs would be the most important part of getting a spot in the Navy. During the next year, the scale that he had purchased and kept in his room dipped a little each day.

One of the added perks of losing so much weight was that girls began to notice him again. One afternoon Evan was walking by the church when he was stopped by a few men standing outside. They were crowded around large black boxes, looking sweaty and tired. Next to them there stood a pretty young girl holding a clipboard.

"Hey man, would you be able to help us? We are trying to take this equipment into the church for a charity fundraiser tonight. We could use an extra set of hands with this box."

Evan shrugged, "This one?" He walked over to the box, bent down, and picked it up effortlessly. Their jaws dropped. "Where do you want it to go?" he asked. They silently pointed into the church. Evan carried the box into the church and looked around as he entered. It was weird being inside a church after so long. Somehow though, it felt right being there. When he walked back out, the girl with the clipboard approached him. "Hi, I'm Sarah," she said shyly. "That was amazing what you did back there."

"Lifting that box? That was nothing."

Sarah smiled at him. "It was pretty amazing," she said.

The two teens began hanging out together over the next couple of weeks. She invited him to go to church with her, and he did. At first, he saw it as an excuse to be with her. It wasn't long before he realized that the people in the church were one big family. He could tell that they would give him the shirt off their backs if he had asked. There was Blake, his youth minister, who he felt he could go to for anything. And then there was his preacher, Joshua, who soon became like a second father to him. He wondered what it would have been like if he had people like them around him when Jake had passed away. Although there was no changing the past now, Evan knew that Sarah, and by extension, her church, would end up changing his life for the better. The one thing still holding him back in life was his gang of friends who seemed to be looking for new ways to cause trouble every day.

"Hey Evan," his friend Andrew called out to him one day while he and the gang were circled around in the parking lot, swigging from a bottle of whiskey. "That Sarah girl you're seeing holds a lot of fundraisers at the church right."

"Yeah," said Evan uneasily. "What about it?"

Andrew shrugged, smirking slightly. "I was just thinking that they must make a lot of money from those fundraisers. And being a church and all, they must be really trusting of their neighbors. So trusting in fact, that I bet it wouldn't be hard to break in and steal some of that money."

"Great idea!" one of the other boys in the group chimed in.

Evan stood up straight. "No Andrew, that's not a great idea."

Andrew walked up to Evan, his eyes narrowed. "Oh really? What will you do about it?"

At that moment, Evan wanted nothing more than to punch Andrew in the face. He stood silently for a few seconds, contemplating his next move, before he finally decided to turn around and walk away.

"You're leaving?" Andrew yelled after him? "Fine, then don't come back! Anyone else who wants to leave can go with him!"

To Evan's surprise, he began to hear more footsteps behind him. He turned to see who they were. Martin and a girl, Hannah, followed close behind him.

"Forget those losers," Evan told Martin, "Let's go."

From that moment on, nothing stood in Evan's way to a better life. Martin, Hannah, and Evan became inseparable. Martin became like

Evan's brother. While he was in weight class doing leg presses, Martin would sit next to him sipping on water and watching him with awe.

"Add more," Martin would always say. Sure enough, Evan would add fifty more pounds to each side and keep lifting, barely breaking a sweat. One day, Martin kept adding more and more weights, trying to get Evan to reach his breaking point. The other students in the class began to gather around, cheering him on. After Evan completed fifty repetitions of four-hundred pounds, Martin added even more weight. Evan squeezed his legs, his teeth clenching.

"1.....2....3...."

The rest of the class looked on in shock as Evan kept lifting the heavy weights. They began counting along with him.

"78....79....80!" The bell rang loudly, signaling the end of the class. They all cheered loudly, clapping him on the back as Martin poured a large bottle of water down Evan's face. Evan's heart raced. He could see himself in just a few years, bench-pressing even more weight with his fellow sailors in the Navy. He smiled widely. In that moment, Evan felt unstoppable.

As he lay in the ditch, Evan opened his eyes and looked around in a daze. When he looked down at his leg and saw it bloody and mangled, he began screaming. "I can't feel my leg!" With a sinking feeling, he began to realize what had just happened; he had been hit by a car, and whoever had done it, had left him to die in this ditch alone. As he heard the sounds of other cars passing by, he became very worried and scared. How would he ever get out of here? Would he ever be found?

After what seemed like hours, Evan decided he had to do something. His legs were now useless, so he used his arms to drag himself toward the road. The fact that most of his body had gone completely numb with pain was a good thing, because it somehow allowed him to pull himself up to the top of the ditch. When he got to the side of the road, he began to wave wildly.

"Help me! Help me!" Evan yelled frantically before passing out.

The next sound he remembered was the wailing of sirens. The policeman jumped out of his car, and knelt near Evan.

"What happened here?" He asked.

Evan couldn't speak. He was shaking too badly and he felt dizzy and light-headed. As Evan began to fall in and out of consciousness, he was only faintly aware of what was going on around him. He heard more sirens. Soon, there were more people bustling around him, shining a light in his eyes, and pulling him onto a stretcher. After a few minutes of this, he heard the voice of another young man, sounding terrified.

"You just left him here?" he heard an angry voice growl.

"I came back though, I came back," he heard the boy say. "It's not my fault; he threw himself in front of my car! He tried to kill himself!"

Evan opened his mouth to protest, but still couldn't say anything. He closed his eyes in defeat, and the world went dark around him.

The ambulance headed toward Vanderbilt Hospital. Within a few minutes, Evan arrived in the emergency department and I rushed to meet him and assess the situation. I knew right away that it was bad. His leg was completely mangled and oozing blood.

After seeing Evan and as they rolled him to the operating room, I went to meet his family. Deep inside me I was very worried as this was my first year in practice and one of the worst injuries I had encountered. As I talked to Evan's father I assured him I would do everything in my power to save his son's life and limb.

Evan was in critical condition. Not only was the artery in his leg severely lacerated, his veins were congested and preventing blood flow. The vascular surgeons and I quickly began operating on him. After several attempts, the vascular surgeons were finally able to provide blood flow to his artery, but it was very difficult. His condition began to stabilize, and we all breathed a sigh of relief. We stabilized his leg that night but I was very concerned that he was going to lose his leg given the long period of time it went without blood.

I met with Evan's parents in his room right after the surgery. When I told them that there was a good chance that we would have to amputate Evan's leg, his mother's face turned pale.

"It's my fault," she whispered, "I shouldn't have let him out of the car. I should have driven him back home."

I touched her on the shoulder reassuringly and she embraced

me and started to cry. I told her I would do everything in my power to help Evan and her family. In these moments it was difficult to not become emotional as I very much understood what this meant; Evan was her son. While Evan and his mother had maintained a distant relationship, this would bring them closer.

Later that afternoon, Evan became alert for the first time since the accident. He looked around the room at the strangers surrounding him.

"Hi honey, it's mom. Do you recognize me?"

Evan blinked, looking confused. "What happened?"

His mom hesitated, her eyes tearing up. "We've got bad news. You went for a run, and you were hit by a car. You must have run about two miles in about fifteen minutes based on where they found you. Your leg was badly damaged. There's a chance you won't be able to walk again."

Evan looked more confused than before. "Wait a second, you're telling me that I ran that fast?" To everyone's surprise, Evan smiled and added, "Way to go out with a bang."

The next day, we performed another surgery to clean out Evan's wounds and evaluate whether his leg could be saved. The artery that the vascular surgeons repaired looked good, and the swelling in his muscles had decreased. This meant there was still a chance we could potentially save his leg.

That evening, Hannah and Martin arrived at the hospital. Evan had just returned from surgery, looking groggy. "Does he know who we are?" Hannah asked Evan's mother. Without saying a word, Evan lifted his hand and threw up a peace sign at his friends. Martin began crying. His two friends stayed with Evan for the rest of the night.

Sarah came to visit Evan the next morning. Her eyes were red and her face was covered with tears. Although Evan loved being finally able to see his girlfriend, he knew that his parents didn't approve of their relationship. One of the worst things about living in a small town is that every family had a history, and not all of them were good. Sarah and Evan's families were involved in a bitter feud that went back generations, and the tension in the room was intense when she was there. Over time, Sarah's visits began to become less and less frequent. As much as it pained Evan to see her go, he knew he had to focus on fighting to save his leg.

A few days after his surgery, I took Evan into the operating room to assess his leg for a third time and to wash out his wounds. Things weren't looking too good. I sighed deeply, quietly predicting what was coming next. As I laid in bed that night and stared at the ceiling unable to sleep, I thought about how I would tell Evan the news. He was so young and had his entire life in front of him. I started to play the entire case back in my head as I always did; could I have done anything differently?

The next morning, I went to Evan's room and sat down by his side. We immediately started to talk about his prognosis and I told Evan I was worried about his leg and that I was not sure it could be saved at this point.

Evan felt his body go numb. He knew what that meant; his dream of joining the military would be over. "Well, here's the question," he began. "If I keep my leg, am I going to be able to walk again, or run again?" He then finally asked the question that he had wanted to ask the entire time. "Will I be able to join the military?" He asked, his voice quivering.

I grabbed his hand in mine and looked him in the eye and told him that we needed to focus on what was before us. I understood how overwhelming this was to a bright young man who had his whole life in front of him. I convinced him to give us some more time to see what would happen and that I would fight together with him until the end. I think that in that moment, this is what Evan needed to hear, he simply wanted to know that I understood what he faced and that I would stand with him.

We sat together in silence for the next few minutes.

Finally he nodded and said, "Fine, a few more days."

For the next few days, Evan underwent numerous surgeries where we washed out his leg and prepared it for flap coverage. Later that week, I took Evan to the operating room and prepared for cleaning his wounds once again. As soon as I removed his bandages, a foul odor wafted through the air. There was pus all over his tibia, and the wound above his femur had partially burst open. Liquid was oozing all over his leg.

I started to examine more carefully knowing fully well what I would find. As I expected, the skin around his tibia had almost completely died off. His muscle was swollen and everything was dead. I had promised Evan that he could make the final call. With a heavy heart, I told the rest of my surgical team to close up his leg as I went to find Evan's father. As I walked into the waiting area, he took one look and knew what was coming next. Together we discussed how best to talk with Evan.

Later that day when Evan woke up I went to his room and delivered the news that he would need an amputation. These conversations are never easy and I always feel like my heart is breaking as I explain to my patient. But as we sat together I assured Evan that he had his whole life ahead of him and that he would walk again with a prosthesis. I told him I would be by his side and that he would make it through.

He took a deep breath. "Okay. Let's do it," he said, holding back tears.

We scheduled his amputation for the next day and Evan was barely able to sleep that night. He knew that along with his leg, he was also losing his dream of joining the Navy. It was the one thing he wanted more than anything in life. What was the point of living now?

The day of his amputation, Pastor Joshua came to visit Evan, bringing with him a large group of Evan's friends from church and a large pile of letters.

"We wrote you letters so you'd have something to read the next few days that you're here," Pastor Joshua said with a smile. "We know this next step is going to be tough, but you'll get through it," he said, squeezing his shoulder.

Pastor Joshua led everyone in a hymn as they huddled around Evan's bed. For the first time in weeks, Evan felt a huge weight being lifted off his shoulders as a wave of calmness swept over him.

Evan lay awake in his bed, gazing at the dark silhouette of his mother sleeping in the chair next to him. After his amputation, Evan stayed in the hospital for another five days for monitoring. Tonight was his first night back home, and he couldn't fall asleep. His parents were taking turns sleeping in his room. "If you need me, just wake me up," his mother said as she settled into the armchair next to his bed. But as Evan lay in the bed, trying to get used to the fact that one of his legs wasn't there, he knew it would be a long night. He sighed in frustration. His mother, who was still awake, reached out and held his hand.

The next morning, Evan realized how much more difficult things were going to get. As he went to leave the bathroom, he suddenly lost his balance and fell, directly onto the stub of his amputated leg. He howled in pain. Having heard the scream, his dad arrived quickly, pounding on the locked door. Evan slid his way toward the door and reached up and opened it. His dad bent down and with a large grunt, picked Evan up off the floor.

"Dad, wait! I'm too heavy for you!"

Without saying a word, his dad carried Evan to the living room and laid him down on the couch. There were tears in his father's eyes.

If there was one good thing that came from this entire ordeal following his accident, it was realizing how much his mother and father loved him. He also felt that same love and dedication from Martin, Hannah, and of course, his church family. The medical bills were starting to pile up. Although he received some financial support from the driver who had hit him, who he later found out was a recent high school grad, just like himself, it was his church that seriously stepped up to the plate. They began planning a benefit to pay the hospital bills and to help Evan get a prosthetic. But before he could begin walking with it, he still had months left in his wheelchair. Martin and Hannah also did everything they could to help Evan during this time.

"Come to my birthday party tonight," Martin requested a few weeks after Evan had been discharged from the hospital. "I'll set up a ramp so you can get into the backyard for the bonfire."

"I'll come if I feel up to it, if I'm not too tired," Evan answered. The truth was, Evan didn't feel like doing anything these days. The military was the only thing he wanted to do when he grew up. It was the one thing that could get him out of town and he felt this accident had taken away his only dream. He knew he had to find something else and move on, but there was nothing else he wanted to do more than serve in the military. He thought back to the poster he had seen his sophomore year, when he was still reeling from Jake's sudden death. This time, he had God, his church, and his friends – all of whom he trusted would never leave his side.

Evan rolled out of his room and said to his mother, "Mom, can you take me to Martin's? It's his birthday."

When Martin saw Evan's car pull into the driveway, he jumped up from his front porch with excitement. "Evan's here!" Martin called out to everyone. He helped him scoot up the porch and to the backyard, where he, Hannah, and Evan sat and talked for hours into the night.

The next few months were hard for Evan. I was a little concerned about him bearing weight on his leg, so he stayed in his wheelchair for a while longer, and after that, he used a walker while becoming familiar with his prosthetic. He took solace in being able to go to church, where he went without fail every week. The accident had caused tension between him and Sarah, and the feud between their families just made things worse. The two decided to take some time apart. By now, however, Evan's ties to the church were not part of Sarah's life. When he listened to the sermons, he felt as if he could muster up the strength to push himself forward, to be the Evan who previously had legs of pure muscle, even if he no longer had both of them.

On Thanksgiving, while the rest of his family was gathered at his house for dinner, Evan knew it was finally time to take his first steps on his own. He pushed his walker to the side and began walking. Before he knew it, he had walked from one side of the living room to the other. He began to walk back and forth, his smile widening every time.

"Hey everyone! Look, Evan's walking!" His dad called out to the family. They all rushed over and gathered around.

Evan beamed back at him. "I did it dad. I can do it."

"I always knew you could, son," his dad replied, his eyes brimming with tears. Evan's grandfather walked up to him and put his hand on his shoulder. "You know grandson, I've had a lot of friends who had lost one of their limbs in the war. And what I learned from those experiences is that the one way you can really defeat a man is by taking away one of his limbs. That's the worst hell you can put him through. But you, you're a fighter."

Evan knew his grandfather was right. Losing his limb didn't mean his life was over. Losing his limb was just another challenge God had given him because He knew Evan could take it. Well then – challenge accepted.

From that moment on, Evan didn't let anything stop him. Before long, it was spring, and Hannah, Martin, Evan, and the rest of their friends finally made it out to Montgomery Bell State Park. As they swam, Evan had to stroke twice as hard with his arms and one leg in order to keep up with the others. Together, they swam up to a tall bluff which stood fifteen feet high above the water. Two long ladders hung treacherously off the bluff, daring swimmers to climb up and jump.

"Let's climb up and jump!" Hannah said excitedly. Evan looked up to the bluff nervously. "Don't worry Evan," Martin said. "We're not going to ask you to climb with us."

"Why not?" answered Evan. "It looks fun."

"It's just one of those things," Martin said uneasily. "We don't want you to get hurt."

Floating in the river, Evan watched as his friends took turns climbing up the ladder. Once they all got to the top, they stood around and looked at each other. Evan smirked. He could tell they were all too scared to be the first one to make the jump. He took a deep breath and began to swim toward the rope.

From the top of the bluff, Martin looked over the edge of the cliff to the deep water below. When he didn't see Evan, he panicked. "Where's Evan?" he cried.

"You mean that guy?" One of the other guys standing on the bluff asked, pointing down toward the ladder.

There was Evan, climbing up, slowly but surely.

"Evan, what are you doing? You're going to get hurt!" Hannah said as she helped him climb over the edge of the bluff.

Evan stood up and smiled. "Too late, I'm already up here. The only way I'm getting down is jumping." He looked at his two best friends "Will you guys jump with me?"

Martin and Hannah smiled knowingly at Evan. "Let's do this," they said in unison.

Evan stood at the corner of the bluff, high above the deep blue-green river. He took one more side-long glance at Martin and Hannah. Then, at the same time, they all closed their eyes, and jumped.

Evan could have allowed the anguish over the loss of his leg to destroy his life; but he didn't. As he had done time and time again he utilized his faith in God and the compassion of his family and friends to propel him forward.

Progress Notes on Evan

Evan will soon be going back to school to study psychology or history. He dreams of becoming a psychologist and helping soldiers suffering from PTSD. He has moved into his own house and is recovering well. With the aid of a prosthesis he is walking again. He has gone on several more adventures with his friends, including trips to Florida and North Carolina.

Brianna

Their names echoed across the top of the hill. "Brianna-Alyssa-Lauren-Roger!" As usual, the names of the four siblings were strung together as if they were all one person. The other kids laughed. "Your mom's calling," they teased. Brianna's cheeks turned red with embarrassment.

"She probably just wants us to come in and find the TV remote," Roger muttered under his breath. The four of them began running up the hill toward their house at the end of the road. It seemed like their mom never ran out of ways to embarrass them. Every afternoon, she would drive up to their school in their old, raggedy car with a giant smoke cloud trailing behind her. Brianna was too humiliated to sit in the front, but her mother always insisted.

Brianna couldn't help but be jealous of the other kids in the neighborhood. About half were her close friends, and the rest were her cousins. In fact, the last time she counted, there were twenty-three cousins from her dad's side in their school. Even though they were all in the same family, some of her cousins were better off financially than she was. She often wondered how her parents and siblings had gotten to this point, down such a different road from many of her relatives.

Her dad worked in another town and was very seldom home. It seemed that lately he was coming home less and less. Sometimes it felt like all she had was her mom, who looked more and more tired every day when she got home from her two jobs. When her father was home, the usual singing and laughing they did with their mom became replaced by bitter arguments and profound tension. She wondered if there'd be a day when her dad would stop coming home at all.

When they heard their mom call their names, they went running and reached their house where their mother was impatiently standing outside the door with her hands on her hips.

"Where have you been? You know we have church first thing in the morning."

"Of course," Roger said with a sigh as he entered the house. "When have we not?"

Their mom looked at him sternly. The four of them always complained about church, but in the end, they couldn't imagine their life without it. It seemed like they practically lived there. All their friends and family went to the same church and every week they had another activity planned with their youth group. This Friday was skate night, and next week they were traveling to a nearby town with their youth chorus group for a performance.

Brianna knew that in the morning, she'd see her Sunday school teacher who would give them all little boxes of raisins. Then she would see Anna, an elderly woman at their church, who would give them each candy bars. When they'd come home, she and all the other kids would change out of their nice Sunday school clothes and play kickball until the street lights grew dim and the familiar call from their mother would ring through the streets once again. The predictable routine made her feel safe, and her family made her feel happy.

When Brianna began high school, her life took a turn for the worse. By then her dad had one foot out the door, and the fights between her parents became even more bitter.

"So you're getting a divorce?" Roger asked his mother, unable to hide the sadness in his voice. "Not a divorce, a divorce is more than I can afford. He's just leaving. It'll be just us now."

"What are we going to do," Brianna asked with panic. "Where will we get money?"

"Don't you worry, we've never had much, and hopefully I'll be able to keep a roof over our heads."

Brianna needed to trust in her mother that everything would be fine. School was a good distraction and she was taking a cosmetology class that she loved. Ruby, one of the women at her church who worked at a local salon, began to take Brianna to work with her and Ruby's clients loved her. Even though she helped out only as a shampoo tech, she could see herself being a hair stylist for the rest of her life. The extra money she received from Ruby was an added bonus, especially with the way things were going at home. She knew her mom was having a hard time making ends meet. Still, she didn't know how bad it actually was until her mom spoke the very words she had always feared.

"The bank is taking the house," her mom said, tears streaming down her face.

"What are we going to do? Where will we all go?" Roger asked with panic.

"I don't know, but I'll figure something out."

Brianna's family was now facing homelessness for the first time in her life. In order to have a roof over their heads, the family was separated. Her mother went to stay at her aunt's house with Brianna's two youngest sisters. Roger went to live with their grandparents. But Brianna desperately didn't want to leave her neighborhood. It was her home, the remnants of her childhood. She felt she was growing up too fast too soon. It wasn't long before news of them being kicked out of their house spread through church.

"You can stay with me," Preacher Strickland told Brianna at church that Sunday. "We're your family too," he said. Brianna was relieved. Preacher Strickland lived in Park Wood, which was close to her current neighborhood. Now that she had a place to stay, she continued to pray for the rest of her family.

Her parents were still not divorced, and with her dad's income, they were not eligible for public assistance. Over the course of the next few weeks, her mother was able to get a legal separation and re-applied for public assistance, which was approved. They were on welfare and food stamps, but there was only so much they could afford for rent. Her mother kept searching for a place to live with hopes she could soon bring her family back together.

"God has answered our prayers!" She exclaimed one day. "I found a house for us to rent. With help from the state we can stay there for as long as we want. And it's close by, so you'll get to stay in your same school."

Brianna was ecstatic. Her family was finally reunited. Their new home was immediately full of song and laughter. Times were tough, but at least they had each other. Brianna went back to working at the hair salon with Ruby. She was glad to have a way to help support her family and for the rest of high school, hair styling became her passion and her dream. Roger graduated high school and moved back with his grandparents to go to college. Brianna, however, wanted to stay with her family for as long as she could and help support them. One of the perks of their new house was they were able to stay in their school, which was mostly attended by kids living in the nicer neighborhoods in Nashville. Every week when she went to the grocery store with her food stamps, she would see the Mercedes and the Cadillacs lined up in the parking lot. Her mind flashed back to their rusty old car, and how embarrassed she felt getting into the front seat in front of all her friends. She didn't want her sisters to have to go through that for the rest of their lives, so she began giving them whatever money she would make from the hair salon so they wouldn't have to ask their mom for money.

She knew how embarrassing it was for her mom to go down to the state agency and talk to case workers. "They talked to me like I was nothing," her mother would say when she came home from the agency.

Brianna was determined to support her family in any way she could. After she graduated, she began working a second job, at a fast food restaurant. At the same time, she attended beauty school where she would be able to get a license and work full time at the salon. Her mom began collecting used glass bottles and selling them to make whatever extra income she could. When Brianna got her check at the end of the week, she gave her sisters a portion of whatever she made.

"The one thing I ask," She would say before she handed them the money "is that we respect each other. We're sisters, and we take care of each other. Remember that."

By the end of the year, Brianna had successfully obtained her license and was able to work full time at the salon. "You have so much potential," Ruby said after seeing the styles she'd practice on the mannequin wigs lining the shop. "You should begin competing in hair styling contests." Brianna was nervous, but she happily agreed. Soon, she and Ruby began traveling around the state to different hair shows. Ruby wasn't the only one who loved Brianna's work, other people across the state would look at her styles and say, "That girl's got something."

At the competitions, usually with more than 100 young women competing, Brianna would consistently end up winning second or third place. Her winnings sparked something within herself, and she began to feel serious about her future at the hair salon. With the girls at the salon, she began holding her own hair shows, the very first to ever take place in Nashville. New clients began visiting her salon from across the city. Her earnings far surpassed what she thought she would ever make doing something she was so passionate about. In stark contrast, her mother continued to struggle financially. She began to wonder if it would be worth it to go back to school, but she knew there was little hope she could afford that. After all, the family was still on welfare.

"Go back to school, mom," Brianna urged her. "I'll help take care of the girls." Brianna continued to work hard at the salon and live with her mother and younger siblings. Still only eighteen years old, she went from working eight hours a day to sixteen hours. Styling was her passion and she knew her new career meant that she would be able to stay with her family and to help them survive financially. As long as she had them, she was happy, but she knew there was only so much she could do. The owners of the house in which they were living in Bordeaux, a Nashville suburb, told them they were thinking of selling the property and they offered to sell it to Brianna and her family for cheap, but it was still way more than they could afford.

"I feel like I can barely keep a roof over my family's heads," her mother said with tears in her eyes. "I really don't know what to do this time."

By now, Roger had moved out of his grandparent's house and into the house where their late great aunt had lived. It was a large, decrepit old house built by their great grandfather, who happened to know nothing about construction. The doors were all different sizes, and there weren't any closets. It currently stood in the middle of the ghetto, and that was the last place Brianna's mother wanted to move her family. And yet, it seemed they had no other choice.

Brianna, her mother, and her sisters moved into the house with Roger. The upstairs was too cramped to fit them all, so she and her sisters stayed downstairs in tiny rooms that were barely big enough for a bed. It felt like they were living in a haunted house, and Brianna knew they had reached a new low. At all hours of the day, there were noises from outside their house – hollering, gunshots, and sirens.

When she'd walk down the street, she'd see drug deals taking place in the open. She was terrified about what could happen to her family.

Every day, Brianna and her family would continue to pray to God to watch over them. She knew this was just another challenge her family had to face together. As the months went by, and Brianna and her family remained safe in their new neighborhood, she began to feel more at ease in their new home. When she came home at the end of the day and locked the door behind her, she would forget about all the danger and violence that was happening just outside.

Brianna lived in the old house for nearly a year, until she turned nineteen. At that point, like many people her age, she was overcome by a strong desire to gain her own independence and move away from her family. She decided to move in with a friend who lived in a college town a few hours outside of Nashville. It was there where she met Owen, who was a student at the university. It was love at first sight for Brianna, and the two of them began dating. The rest was all a blur. By the end of the year, they were married. Soon after the wedding, they moved to his home town of Indianapolis.

Brianna and Owen's first few years together were full of wedded bliss. It didn't take long, however, for Brianna to realize how hard married life could actually be. She didn't realize how much she still needed her family until she was hundreds of miles away from them. Brianna and Owen fought constantly, and she began to get the sinking feeling that maybe she had gotten married too young. She was desperate to make it work and she devoted her time and energy to the marriage. She gave up on her dreams of becoming a professional hair stylist to get a more stable, nine to five job working in an office. It wasn't her passion, but it paid the bills.

Brianna ended up staying in Indianapolis with Owen for sixteen years. During this time, she broke off all her ties with her family. She didn't want them to know how miserable she was in her new life. But no matter how much she tried to make it work with Owen, neither of them were happy with their lives together. Eventually, Brianna came to the realization that her marriage with

Owen was never going to work. When she was thirty-five years old, Brianna decided to file for divorce.

After the divorce, Brianna had no reason to stay in Indianapolis. She returned to Nashville, where she found a job working as a receptionist at a large medical company.

Four more years passed by in Nashville, where she lived alone in a one bedroom apartment. She remained hopeless and disillusioned about her future and disappointed about her past. She began to pour all of her energy into her work. She barely slept at night, and had to drink several energy drinks throughout the day to stay awake.

Now thirty-nine years old and divorced, Brianna was terrified that she would end up unmarried and being alone for the rest of her life. The hardest part of this ordeal was realizing that she would probably never have kids. Although she felt isolated in her new life, she didn't want to burden her family with the deep depression she felt enveloping her more and more every day. She learned how to put on a fake smile and mask her true feelings. Her mother was the closest person who could relate to what she was going through, having been married young and divorced herself.

She talked with her mom the most, and that was maybe 10 minutes a week. Brianna barely talked to her siblings. Alyssa and Lauren were both married and had kids of their own. They didn't know what it was like to be divorced and alone.

One morning, Lauren called Brianna. To her surprise, Brianna actually picked up. "I don't even know where you live, Brianna," her sister Lauren said during their phone conversation.

That's exactly what Brianna had wanted. She had fallen off the face of the earth, and she did so intentionally. She was the oldest sister and was accustomed to taking care of her family, but now she knew that she had to take care of herself and get her own mental state in control before she could involve them back in her life. But for some reason that morning, she felt she needed her sister more than ever. They ended up talking on the phone for more than an hour.

"My biggest fear in life is that something will happen to me and no one will know. I fear that I'm going to die alone," Brianna told her sister over the phone, her voice quivering.

Brianna knew she couldn't keep living like this, alone and pushing all those who loved her further away. Earlier that week, her friend Leah from work had invited her to drive to Florida with her and her daughter. Brianna had taken her up on her offer, thinking that it was about time she had a vacation with the hope that it would help lower the stress in her life. They would be leaving that afternoon, as soon as Brianna and Leah got off work.

Brianna left the office and began driving home but found herself struggling to stay awake. As usual, she had barely slept the night before. Brianna's eyelids became heavier and heavier with each passing second. Leah and her daughter would be at Brianna's house in an hour, ready to head off on their road trip. But as a wave of exhaustion began to overcome Brianna, she wondered if she had the energy to take this long trip with them.

Brianna dozed off for a few seconds. Her hands slipped off the steering wheel, turning it ever so slightly to the left as they did. Her car swerved across the double yellow lane and slammed head on into a large truck. Brianna's car crumpled like a piece of paper in mere seconds by the force of the collision. Her car skidded to a halt on the side of the road as it burst into flames.

Bystanders near the scene were in shock at the horrific scene. Coincidently, Brianna's second cousin from her dad's side, Joseph, who went to her church was driving the truck she had hit. Her uncle's brother-in-law, Anthony, was two cars behind her. He took one look at the woman inside the car sprawled across the seat, unrecognizable with her face bloodied, and knew that she must be dead. Emily, a nurse who lived in the house next to the accident ran to the mangled car to see if she could help. As she stood a few feet from the flaming car with the rest of the crowd, she could see right away that both of Brianna's legs and her arm were severely contorted. She couldn't tell if Brianna had suffered any severe internal injuries, however, which would mean the difference between her being dead or alive.

The passersby on the side of the road tried to help, but the burning flames obstructed them from reaching Brianna, whom they presumed must already be dead from the horrible crash. Luckily, within just a few minutes, an ambulance arrived on the scene. The medics extinguished the fire, and quickly ran to her side. One of them checked Brianna's pulse.

"She's alive," he said in disbelief.

They carefully extracted her from the burning vehicle and laid her on a stretcher. Brianna's eyelids fluttered. "What happened?" she asked, her voice slurred.

"Ma'am, could you tell us your name?"

"Brianna Johnson," she murmured. She recited a telephone number to them and asked if someone would call her mother.

The medics wheeled her into the ambulance. Sirens blaring, they rushed her to the emergency room of Vanderbilt Hospital. The medic told the doctors that she was conscious and talkative for the entire trip. One of the bystanders took the number and called Brianna's mom.

Upon arrival at the hospital she was rushed to the operating room. One of the trauma surgeons, Dr. Mark Lewis, assessed her wounds. She had a high energy fracture of her left thigh bone and her right lower leg had been shattered and she had also fractured her spine. Dr. Lewis was worried that her right leg would eventually need to be amputated. He fixed her left femur and temporarily stabilized her right leg.

By the time she came out of surgery, Brianna's entire family had arrived. The emergency department was crowded with Brianna's siblings, nieces, nephews, cousins, and her mother. There were about thirty-five of them all together. One of the nurses walked up to them once the surgery was over. They huddled round her with anticipation.

"She just came out of surgery, and her condition is stabilizing," the nurse said as she looked with disbelief at the large crowd, "You can see her, but," she held up her hands in warning, "only two people at a time."

Brianna's mother and Alyssa were the first taken to her room in the trauma unit. The moment Brianna's mother saw her lying in her bed, hooked up to the machines and bruised all over her body with her arms and legs in large bandages, she began to cry. It was also shocking for Alyssa to see her like that; Brianna, their strong, independent sister, lying helpless in the hospital bed fighting for her life.

When Brianna woke, she looked out at her mother and sister in a daze. When she saw her mother's face, tears formed in her eyes. "Mom," she said quietly. "What happened to me?"

Over the next few days, Brianna kept going in and out of consciousness. Every time she did, she'd forget where she was and how she got there. She remained bed-ridden, unable to eat or even use the bathroom by herself. During this time, Brianna's family would take turns coming to see her. When they visited her room, they would walk by other victims of motorcycle wrecks and car accidents. Many of them would be there one day and their room would be completely empty the next day. Every time this happened, they said a prayer.

Around this time Joseph, her second cousin who was driving the truck that she had hit, came to see Brianna. He had snuck into her room while she was asleep to see how she was doing. Brianna's mother told him that she was still recovering.

"In fact, she was worried about you," she said. "One of the first things she asked me was if anybody else was hurt."

"You can let her know I am just fine," Joseph said. "And I'll come back to see her when she's better."

Over the next few days, Brianna had several more surgeries. She had also suffered severe burns in the crash. Now that we had taken care of her more emergent orthopedic injuries, she continued to be treated for her burns.

Brianna's mother and her sister Lauren took turns staying with her. They made sure she wasn't alone for one second. Occasionally, Brianna would open her eyes and look around in panic, wondering where she was. In those moments, Lauren or her mother would take her hand and hold on until she fell back asleep.

A week after the accident Dr. Lewis handed Brianna's care over to me. He was very concerned about the right leg and the ability to save it. I met and talked with Brianna and her family for an hour about the path ahead. I explained there would be multiple surgeries and that we would do everything in our power to save her leg. I could tell that Brianna and her mother were scared and I asked them to trust me.

A few days later, I took Brianna to the operating room and I immediately saw that her badly fractured leg would need special care and that it would be a tricky surgery to complete. Six hours later, we were done.

After the surgery, I was still worried about her eventual recovery and I consulted with several of my colleagues. I was worried that eventually she would lose her leg or at best would need to undergo further surgeries to save it. As disheartening as it was, I knew I had to tell her the risks. Brianna closed her eyes and nodded. "I understand," she said softly. "All I can do now is pray." We prayed together.

Brianna like so many of my patients was an incredible individual and a Tennessean who had worked hard her entire life to provide for her family and to rise from the shackles of poverty – she demonstrated the power of the American Dream in Tennessee. I could never understand why patients like Brianna found themselves in harm's way but as my Pastor Stephen Handy told me, it was not my place to understand.

Brianna remained in the hospital for three more weeks. She was eventually moved back to the trauma unit. At any one time, there were more than 10 people there, waiting to have their turn to visit her room. All the cousins she had grown up with were there, even though she hadn't seen them in years. Along with them were aunts and uncles, church members, her pastor, her friends from the hair salon she had worked with twenty years earlier, and her current coworkers.

"I've never seen so many people here for one person!" her nurse exclaimed.

As cousin Joseph had promised, he returned to the hospital to see Brianna. This time around, Joseph brought his family and they all sang together. Brianna felt relieved to finally meet the man who she had hit and to see that he was okay.

Brianna remained in a back brace, due to her spinal fractures, during this period of recovery and her nurses had to come in on a regular basis and flip her back and forth in the bed. She was completely helpless. The trauma, plastic surgery, and orthopedics teams came in every day to update her on our treatment plans. Lauren and Alyssa began keeping a journal to write down all the different medications she took. At night, Brianna would have nightmares and thrash about in her bed.

"You're fine, you're fine," her sister would assure her, waiting at her side until she fell back asleep.

After the swelling in her ankle went down, I was able to perform a second surgery on her leg. Even if the surgery went well, she still had a very high risk of infection and amputation. That surgery took another six hours, and piece by piece we put her leg back together.

I met with Brianna and her family in her room after surgery and I told them I was hopeful about her recovery. They broke down in tears as they held each other. Within a few days, Brianna was discharged to a rehabilitation center.

The move was difficult for Brianna, and she was in an unbearable amount of pain while she waited to be situated in her new home. Luckily she wasn't at the center for too long, and was ready to be discharged within a few weeks.

"What do I do?" she asked her sister Alyssa. "I'm going to lose my job eventually and I'll run out of money."

"Don't worry about that," Lauren responded. "You'll move in with me. It'll be cramped, but we'll manage. It'll be like old times, like at great grandpa's house."

Brianna smiled, "That'll be nice," she said.

Before Brianna's arrival, Lauren made sure everything was ready. A makeshift ramp was built to her new room, which was converted from the family's old den. Alyssa's daughter, Jordan, who had just graduated high school also moved in with Lauren so she could help take care of Brianna.

"There's no way a stranger is going to come in here and take care of my sister," Alyssa had said. "Jordan can take care of her."

"We can't ask her to do that," Brianna had exclaimed. "She just graduated and she'll want to find a job."

"I'll pay her," Lauren said. "Jordan dreams of being a nurse. You can be her first patient."

Tears formed in Brianna's eyes. She was still terrified of what would happen in the long term and wondered if she could ever make a full recovery. To know that her family would be at her side throughout this whole process lifted a heavy weight off her shoulders. Before her accident, Brianna had felt completely and utterly alone.

She had wondered if anyone would even notice if she was gone. Now she knew the answer.

Throughout the next few months, Brianna's family rallied together and made sure she had everything she needed. Jordan diligently cared for her aunt every day. Almost daily, Alyssa would come by with her younger kids, Hailey, Alexis and Jaylen, who adored Brianna. The moment she called for them, they were at her side, driving her around the house in her wheelchair and dispensing her medication for her. Her mother was also at the house, taking care of her as she always had. The most surprising, however, was her father.

Brianna's father had not been present throughout her life. When he heard about her accident, he wanted to do anything he could to help. He came to the hospital every morning and every evening. He even went to the car shop where her car had been stored after her accident. He called her when he reached the shop and saw the car, which was too badly damaged to be repaired. He thought of Brianna sitting in that car when she crashed into the truck, and began to cry. Brianna was stunned. She had never once heard him cry.

Brianna's reunion with her father was one of the most incredibly positive things that had come out of her near life ending trauma. I had seen this time and time again, after sustaining such intense tragedies, many of my patients turned their lives around by repairing broken relationships with their spouses and families and ending addictions to drugs and alcohol.

As the months went by, Brianna's finances began to dwindle. Her sisters came up with the idea of throwing a benefit for her, and Roger wholeheartedly supported the idea. He had learned to make short films and documentaries, and decided he would create one about Brianna's accident and recovery. The family had taken many pictures at the hospital, and Roger had been filming as well. He volunteered: "I'll work on it during the next few weeks and put something together that we can show at the benefit."

"I can make fliers," Alyssa offered. "We'll talk to the pastors at church; they'll help us put something together."

By that weekend, the entire neighborhood was filled with flyers. Their church was buzzing with news of Brianna's benefit and her return to church. She began to feel hopeful for the future. The only thing still weighing on her mind was whether or not her legs would heal. She had continued to see me at the clinic throughout this time and she continued to improve. I was so thankful to God, as was she, that we were able to save both of her legs.

Brianna began to be hopeful for the future and she knew she was lucky to be alive. She realized that this accident could have been a blessing in disguise. It was only after facing such great suffering that she had realized how strong her family's bonds truly were.

When the day of the benefit arrived, Brianna couldn't help but feel nervous. She had pushed so many people out of her life during the last few years since her divorce, she was concerned how bad it would be if nobody showed up. It had been several months since her last surgery, but she was still in a wheelchair. Because of that, she had to be transported in the access ride van.

"Are you ready?" Alyssa asked her before they headed off to the van.

Brianna took a deep breath, "I am," she said.

Alexis, one of her nieces, wheeled Brianna out the front door and Jordan walked beside them. The van was waiting outside. They lowered the ramp for her wheelchair. As Alexis wheeled her down the driveway, without any warning whatsoever, Brianna fell out of the wheelchair and onto the grass, landing on her legs.

"Auntie Brianna!" Alexis exclaimed, picking her up quickly and helping her back into the chair. Brianna looked down at her cast, which was now covered with dirt. She started crying.

"Don't worry Aunt Brianna," Jordan said, "It's just some dirt, I can wipe it off."

Brianna couldn't tell her that it was more than just the dirt she was crying about. Alexis rode with Brianna while her sister and her family drove along in another car. She was overcome with anxiety throughout the ride and once again wondered who would be waiting at the church when she arrived. Her stomach was in knots.

When they were just a few miles away from the church, they passed the scene of a bad accident on the other side of the highway. A car was turned over on its side and several police cars were gathered around, lights flashing. Brianna began sobbing. She thought back to the other patients in the trauma ward. She knew at least a handful of them had suffered car accidents that were not nearly as bad as hers. All of them had died. "Why am I still here, Lord?" she thought, her heart pounding as tears streamed down her face. "Why me, Lord?"

By the time she got to the church and Alyssa opened up the doors of the van, Brianna's eyes were completely bloodshot and her face was streaked with tears.

Alyssa hugged her sister tightly. "Don't worry sis, I'm here," she said, wiping away her tears.

Roger and Lauren came outside to greet their sister. "You're here!" they exclaimed when they saw her. "Everyone's been waiting!"

Brianna took a deep breath. "Do we have to do this?" she asked.

Roger smiled at her, "Just wait until you see," he promised.

Alyssa wheeled Brianna up to the church doors. Roger and Lauren opened the doors on either side and Alyssa wheeled her in. Brianna gasped.

The church was filled with a sea of familiar faces; the cousins she grew up with, her friends from her old salon, her coworkers, and relatives from all over were here. There was Bailey from Detroit, and Keith from St. Louis. As a group, they were smiling widely and clapping as she made her entrance.

The benefit was beautiful. There were bands, speeches, singing, and laughter. As Roger's photos from Brianna's accident were displayed on a large screen, her mother and sisters told her story.

"We're all here because of Brianna's accident, but not all of you have been filled in on the details. For those who don't know this already, laughter is a big part of our lives. So we're going to tell her story, our own way."

As the photos flashed across the screen, Brianna's sisters began sharing her story as the band played. Rather than making it sad and depressing, they put a creative spin on it, making everyone, including Brianna, laugh out loud. Toward the end of the slideshow, they showed a picture of her car from the day of her accident. Anthony, her relative who was on the scene during the accident, had snapped the photo after she was taken away by the ambulance. It was the first time she had seen her car in that state – her windshield had shattered into a million pieces and the car itself was crumpled up to half its actual size. A lump formed in her throat. In that moment, she knew how blessed she was to not only be alive, but to have her family at her side.

Following her story, they played a series of video interviews Roger had conducted with her friends and family.

"What was your first response when you heard about Brianna's accident?" he asked one of their cousins, Shannon.

"Well it was 6:30 on a Wednesday. Of course, most of us had already left for church by then. So when you called, I knew right away something had gone wrong."

Hearing everyone's reactions to her accident was shocking to Brianna. How could she ever have thought at one time that she was alone in this world?

After the video, Joseph came up to the podium. He introduced himself. "Hi everyone, I'm Joseph. I was driving the truck that Brianna hit on the day of her accident."

Brianna's eyes widened. She was very happy and surprised to see Joseph.

"For weeks after the accident, I had nightmares," Joseph admitted. "After Brianna hit my truck and I saw her car crumpled on the side of the road I knew without a doubt that whoever was in that car would surely have been killed. All the other people who were on that road with me, some of whom are here now, believed the same thing. There was no way that whoever was in that car could still be alive." He paused. "And yet here we are today. Seeing how many people are here, I know that somebody was watching over her that day."

While Brianna's injuries were different than those of Aaron, Kristen, Michael, or my other patients in this book, her healing in large part was due to the same factors: her strong faith, family, and the power of the love that came from the community. At so many points in her recovery she could have given up, but her belief in God sustained her, and her friends and family picked her up when she fell down. I felt a kinship with Brianna, because I experienced the same powerful forces in my own life. I understood the gravity of these forces not only as a surgeon but also as a son of two immigrants who sought and then lived the American Dream in Tennessee.

Brianna felt chills go through her body. She knew right away that the Lord must have saved her for a reason. Before her accident, she had barely felt alive. Her family and friends – the people who mattered most to her – were no longer a part of her life at that point. They had been through so much together as children, and she needed something like this to remind herself that they would always be there for her. Maybe, Brianna pondered, the day of the accident wasn't the day she almost died. Maybe it was the day she started living again.

Progress Notes on Brianna

Brianna is doing well. She needed another major surgery on her left thigh which was successful and has now allowed her to walk independently. She is actively involved with her family and is making a documentary about her accident and the road to recovery. She spends a great deal of time volunteering in her church and local community.

Jessica

"Do you feel this?"

Jessica looked up at Dave, tears forming in her eyes.

She answered quietly. "No."

Jessica closed her eyes tightly. It was time to have a conversation with God. "Now look," she said silently in her head. She knew at a time like this, He would be listening. "This isn't fair for mom and dad. Just take me home. Let's go home now."

The siren's blared in the background, but her mind wandered back to Colorado.

With her eyes closed, Jessica imagined her parents as if they were standing right in front of her. Her father had his arms wrapped around her mother, and the majestic mountains and the Colorado sky loomed behind them. It never ceased to surprise her that after fifty-two years of marriage, her parents were still blissfully in love. The thought of them brought back fond memories of her childhood in Colorado.

Jessica grew up in a modest, hardworking family. She was taught from a very young age that in order to succeed, she needed to work hard.

"If you want to make a difference in your life," her folks would always say, "you have to be the one to do it."

Jessica's family loved exploring the great outdoors of Colorado. She loved her new home state of Tennessee, but the one thing that always bothered her was how everyone seemed to hibernate in the winters; just like the brown bears up on Pike's Peak in Colorado Springs. During winters in Colorado her family would pack up their gear and head out to the mountain for skiing.

In the summer, Jessica attended church camp with her neighbors. Spending those hot, lazy summer days reading the Bible and learning about God were the moments when Jessica found her unconditional faith for the Lord. She felt as if He had wrapped His arms around her at a young age, promising to never let go. As a child, her family went to church only during the traditional two or three times a year during the holidays, but it was much different for her now as a grown-up.

As Jessica lay on the ground and reminisced about her childhood, she could almost feel the warm Colorado sunshine on her face. Every weekend, she would explore the great outdoors – from hiking, to skiing, to fishing, and camping in the mountainside with her entire family huddled up into two large tents. Once they had packed up and prepared for these outings and it was time to go, her mother would tell them to jump in the car, and within minutes she and her siblings would chime in with the familiar, "Are we there yet?"

Perhaps their adventurous childhood made it inevitable that Jessica and her brothers would continue to seek out thrills as adults, thrills that too often would bring them to the brink of death. Her oldest brother Josh had always dreamed of being an airline pilot with the freedom to fly anywhere in the world. After a terrible bicycling accident left him with severe head trauma, Josh's dream of learning to fly commercial jets was no longer realistic. When her younger brother Andy was just nineteen years old, he was severely injured in a diving accident. As a result, his spinal cord was severed and he was forced to live the rest of his life as a quadriplegic. Up until this day, only Jessica and her younger sister remained in the same shape and form that God had made them.

As sirens sounded loudly around her, Jessica shed a tear. She knew from Dave's eyes what had just happened to her legs. Her parents didn't need another paralyzed child. Seeing Andy suffer every day was already difficult for them to bear. Jessica knew that if she asked God to spare her parents from suffering, He would listen.

When she was still eighteen, Jessica moved away from her loving home in Colorado to attend a private Christian college in Nebraska. Even though it was heartbreaking to leave her family, she knew God would keep her safe. Her life at the small, quaint school was filled with faith, love, and newfound friends and family.

Jessica's experiences in the real world were not as pleasant. Shortly after college, she began working at a large retail supercenter in Arkansas. From there, she was transferred to Franklin, Tennessee, a small town just south of Nashville. She eventually left her job at the large retail store and found a position working as an administrator in a doctor's office. During staff training, she had the opportunity to travel across the state. No matter where she was - the rolling country sides of Savannah, the lively cities of Memphis and Nashville, or back home in Franklin, Jessica experienced an exuberance of faith that was unmatched anywhere else she had lived.

Her time in the healthcare industry introduced her to two of the most important people she would know in her life. Jansen was a young, Christian woman who worked with Jessica. They developed an instant bond that made them inseparable. Jessica saw immediately that Jansen's loyalty to her faith was mirrored in her friendships.

A few years after she began working in the doctor's office, Jessica met Dave, one of the doctor's patients. As a first responder and an officer for the local fire department, Dave was the type of man who Jessica knew would always keep her safe. Still, she knew that a relationship with Dave wouldn't be appropriate since he was a patient at the office where she worked. Maybe it was the adventurous side of her that led her to take the leap, but before she even knew it, Jessica was in love. After a year of dating, they decided to get married.

Jessica and Dave's relationship was filled with many years of great joy. Unfortunately, after nearly two decades of marriage, they began to grow apart. What were once happy conversations turned into constant arguments. Jessica's job at the doctor's office was also extremely frustrating. She felt a personal connection to the patients who came into the office, but she felt constrained by the endless regulations and red tape that she had to deal with from the large insurance companies.

She left health care and decided to go back to school and earn a cosmetology license with the hopes of being able to open her own upscale salon. It was during cosmetology school that Jessica met Margy. As a loving Christian woman, Margy quickly assumed the role of a protective sister in Jessica's life. With the troubles in her marriage, Jessica knew she could turn to Margy for support.

Although Dave and Jessica would argue nearly every day, both of them had an insatiable thirst for life and adventure. Despite all their differences, they both shared a passion for riding motorcycles. With the wind in her hair, her husband riding closely behind her, they both felt that the sky was the limit. Nothing could stop them. She was in great physical shape and in just a few days, she planned to run her first half marathon. The t-shirt with her marathon runner number was already hanging in her closet.

As Jessica lay there on the ground, she looked into Dave's eyes. She saw the terror in his face as he watched his wife lay nearly lifeless on the pavement. They had their problems before this, but Jessica knew that neither of them would ever be the same after this moment.

Just a few hours earlier, Jessica and Dave were riding to dinner at the local Mexican restaurant. With Jessica in front, Dave followed closely behind her.

After dinner Jessica and Dave set off on their bikes and headed home. In a few miles, they had approached an intersection where the light had just turned green, but as Jessica entered the intersection, a large black SUV driving from the opposite direction started to make a left turn directly in front of her.

With horror, Jessica quickly realized there was another car directly behind her. She was trapped in the intersection with nowhere to go with much-larger vehicles surrounding her on all four sides. In that split-second, she thought of laying her bike down and sliding across the pavement, but she knew if she did that, the car behind her would probably run over her. Instead, she braced herself for the impact.

The large SUV crashed into her left side with incredible force knocking her off the bike. She landed on the hood of the car, smashing her head into the windshield. An unbearable jolt of pain shot up Jessica's left leg as it was hit by the car. For a few seconds, everything went black.

When she opened her eyes, she was somersaulting through the air. Her riding boots and helmet flew off and she landed hard on the pavement. When she fell onto her right side, she heard a sickening crunch in her legs.

Dave was able to avoid the crash and was able to stop. He sat frozen on his bike, watching with disbelief. When he saw Jessica's helmet fly into the air, his stomach lurched. He knew that when a helmet flies off in an accident, there is usually a head inside of it.

Dave immediately jumped off his bike and ran to Jessica. He transformed into first responder mode, assessing the situation and Jessica's wounds. When he saw her look up at him he felt a fleeting sense of relief that all of her was still there.

While Dave tried to stabilize Jessica she had begun her conversation with God. In the meantime, an anxious crowd had begun to form around the two of them. From the distance, Jessica could hear sirens. Strangers bustled and talked loudly around her.

"Oh my God, where is her foot?"

"Is she going to die?!"

"My wife is calling 911."

"Step back – I'm a nurse!"

Jessica felt a hand on her shoulder. A small voice spoke to her softly. "I want to pray for you."

The sirens stopped. She knew the paramedics had arrived.

Jessica had learned much about first responders and medical protocol from Dave. When the ambulance pulled up and Luke and Steve jumped out, she immediately recognized them. She knew nearly every officer in the station and these were two of the younger paramedics who had joined the team several years ago. When Steve and Luke looked over and saw Dave and Jessica, their eyes widened.

"Dave!" Luke cried, "What happened?"

"Car crashed into her on the left side – both of her legs look broken. She is bleeding profusely. She needs to get to a hospital ASAP."

Steve came over to Dave and began pulling him away from Jessica, "I'm sorry Dave, but you need to step back."

As soon as Dave was away from the scene, Steve kneeled near Jessica's legs while Luke moved toward her head, propping her up on his lap. Steve examined her legs. The lower part of her left leg was hanging onto her body by about an inch and a half of skin. Steve became as pale as Jessica was at that moment.

"Don't move," said Luke. "Does anything hurt?"

"My legs," said Jessica, wincing in pain, "It feels like there's hot lava pouring down them."

Luke looked up at Steve with worry. "It's probably her femoral artery – she is bleeding out, fast."

Jessica began to feel dizzy. It took everything in her power to remain conscious. She knew that Dave and Steve must be feeling immense pressure treating an officer's wife. She tried to comfort them.

"You're doing great, guys," she encouraged them. Their faces spun in front of her. She closed her eyes, feeling a darkness overcome her.

"Jessica!" Steve began shaking her. "Jessica, when's you birthday?"

Jessica opened her eyes. "December 8, 1965," she murmured, her eyelids fluttering.

Jessica knew that Steve was trying to keep her conscious to prevent her from going into shock, but she was slowly beginning to fade away.

"Jessica, I'll need to cut your coat," said Luke.

Jessica jerked up. "You can't," she cried. "It's a 100 year Harley Davidson anniversary jacket. Don't worry I can get out of it." She began to wiggle her arms.

"No, Jessica, don't move!" yelled Steve.

"Well cut it on the seams then," she pleaded desperately. "I have a friend who is a seamstress."

"Jessica, I'm sorry."

Jessica heard a large rip, and her heart sank.

While Steve and Luke were freeing Jessica of her clothes, the LifeFlight helicopter from Vanderbilt Hospital was hovering over them.

Todd looked up at one of the other paramedics. "How did they get here so fast?" he asked incredulously.

"I didn't even know anyone called them," he answered. "They must have just been in the area."

"What a weird coincidence," said Steve.

Jessica didn't believe in coincidences. As she looked up at the helicopter, she knew that God was indeed there with her. Suddenly, another jolt of pain shot up Jessica's left leg. Luke looked down at her leg, which was continuing to bleed liberally.

Jessica closed her eyes again, and the sounds around her began to fade away. She laid her head back into Steve's lap. She felt as if she was falling away from the world and into a dark abyss. When she opened her eyes again, it wasn't Steve's lap that she was laying in. It was God's. Jessica's eyes widened. Jesus was kneeling next to her, holding her hand reassuringly. The Holy Spirit floated above them.

"Honey," said Jesus. To her surprise, he had a southern accent. "Honey, you're going to be okay. God's got this. We've got this one taken care of."

Jesus looked up at the sky. Jessica looked up too, at the night stars and the clear, white moon. She knew they were taking her to heaven.

As the LifeFlight chopper landed next to Jessica, Steve, and Todd, the other paramedics began to carry Jessica to the chopper. She didn't take her eyes off Steve's face this entire time. His familiar face kept her calm. It wasn't until she was safely in the chopper that Steve finally left her sight.

When the helicopter arrived at Vanderbilt, the paramedics rushed her into the emergency room. One of the nurses came over with a shot she injected into Jessica's arm. A few seconds after that, everything went black.

Jessica was in very bad shape when I first met her in the emergency room, she had femur fractures on both sides and a badly open fracture of her left lower leg. In situations like this time was of the essence and we got her immediately into the operating room. I went to the waiting area to speak with Dave. As I sat down with him he asked me if Jessica was going to "make it" and I told him that I believed she would. I explained that we would take her to the operating room to stabilize her legs but that I was very worried about her left leg and if it could even be saved.

Dave just looked at me in shock and I stayed silent for a moment. These conversations were never easy and I could tell how scared he was. As I sat there I imagined what it would be like if someone told my wife Maya the same news about me – I wanted to ease his pain in that moment but knew I couldn't.

I walked to the operating room and began the surgery. That day we spent more than six hours putting Jessica's left leg back together. Her leg was contaminated with dirt and I was worried about infection but I believed that we could save it. In the coming days she would require multiple trips to the operating room to repeatedly wash her left leg.

When she woke later that day, it was the first time Jessica realized she was in the hospital. She had no recollection of anything beyond being brought to the emergency room. She looked around the room and saw Dave and Jansen, both laid back in chairs next to her, fast asleep. Seeing Jansen loyally by her side almost made Jessica cry. Both Jansen and Margy knew of the struggles in Jessica's marriage, and they now knew she would need their support more than anything to get through this. Jessica was sure her family would be coming soon to take care of her, because after all, they were obligated. Margy and Jansen weren't. They were there because they chose to love and care for her – she was truly blessed.

As Jessica became more aware of what had happened I came to visit her. As I sat down next to her, I told her about the operations that we had performed and the challenges we faced to save her leg. I quickly figured out that Jessica was a very strong and determined woman who was driven by her faith. She knew with God's help, she would have a fast recovery and that whatever happened was meant to be. She wanted to do everything to save her leg and I was right there with her. As I left her room that day she held her hand in mine and told me that she believed in me and made me promise that I would do my best for her. I assured her that I would. That's just what Jessica does – she brings the best out of people.

Despite their troubles, Dave stayed loyally at Jessica's side during this time. She was heavily medicated so it took a while for the severity of her situation to sink in. Most days, she was nauseous and had immense headaches. There were moments when the unbearable pain would seep through and overcome her entire body and there were times when the memories of what happened to her would come flooding back. She would quickly grab the pen and notebook at her side and begin to write down her thoughts. When she reflected on everything that had happened to her, she never doubted for a second that God was protecting her. Instead of losing her faith, it was magnified the night of the accident while she lay in His lap.

"Jessica, you've been through hell and back," said Margy. She reclined back in the chair next to Jessica. The two of them were watching TV in the hospital room. "There's going to be a lot of pain in your future," she said.

"I don't think so, Margy," said Jessica with a small smile. "I didn't go to hell and back. On that day, I went to heaven and back."

"What do you mean?" asked Margy.

Jessica hadn't told anyone about what she had experienced the night of her accident – she didn't seem to have the right words to explain it. "Let's just say, I was literally knocking on heaven's door."

Margy laughed. "God has blessed you with a spirit of spit and grit," she smiled.

"He has," agreed Jessica. "God has given me such strength that if I needed to move a mountain, I could do it with my own hands."

Two weeks after her initial hospital admission and after multiple surgeries, Jessica was discharged from Vanderbilt and sent to Stallworth Rehabilitation Hospital. I remained worried about her leg but only time would tell. When she was led to the tiny room that seemed to her to be no larger than a broom closet, she reminded herself that God had an amazing sense of humor. A couple of times during the night, Jessica was shuffled off to a new room. During one of those switches, she was led to a room that barely had enough space to fit her bed and a chair for Margy. The two of them laughed uncontrollably as Margy climbed over Jessica's bed to the tiny chair crammed in the corner. When Jessica was treated by grouchy nurses, she found ways to make them laugh.

One week later Jessica came to my clinic with her left leg draining with infection. As I talked to her my heart sank – had we lost the battle to save her leg? But Jessica refused to give up and she wanted to keep fighting to save it. In the coming days we would again go to the operating room multiple times to cleanse her leg. At this point she had lost so much skin and muscle that one of my plastic surgery colleagues transplanted a large piece of muscle from her abdomen to her leg to cover the wound.

Throughout all of the surgeries and all of the uncertainty Jessica remained steadfast and unshaken, in many ways because of the strength of her faith and the love of her family and community. When I would visit Jessica during my rounds, I would be greeted by a large group of people, standing around her with enough balloons and flowers to fill the entire floor.

"We're her friends from church."

"Clients from her salon."

"Brother and sister."

Even more incredible to see was Jessica's constant beaming smile – to me, it was a representation of her unwavering faith and optimism.

In early November, a month after the accident, Dave was finally able to bring Jessica home. Witnessing his wife's accident had scared Dave. Each night before he went to bed, images of that day would pop into his head and follow him into his nightmares. When he'd wake and see Jessica immobilized in her hospital bed in the living room, it was yet another reminder that his nightmares were a reality. Yet, he understood that however difficult this ordeal was for him, it was much worse for Jessica. As hard as it was, he was determined to continue to provide his unconditional support to his wife while she needed him.

Luckily, Dave didn't have to care for Jessica alone. An outpouring of support came from not only Tennessee, but the entire world. Jessica's story had been passed along from church to church. She received messages from Christians in other countries, letting her know that they were praying for her recovery. Ladies groups, Bible classes, youth groups, college kids from churches that Jessica had no knowledge of were offering their assistance in cooking meals, watching her, and taking care of her dog. The Franklin Firefighters Association and the Franklin Noon Rotary built a ramp to Jessica's house for her wheelchair. They remodeled her master bedroom so she would have a roll-in shower. The Tennessee Chiropractic Association held a statewide fund drive to help pay for some of Jessica's medical bills. When Jessica's mother and sister came to stay with her, Jessica was ecstatic. The unwavering support from the community gave Jessica strength. One-hundred days after her accident, Jessica stood for the first time.

In January, Jessica came back to Vanderbilt Hospital for what we had hoped would be her final surgery. She required a bone graft on her lower left leg to replace the bone that had broken off during her accident. The surgery went well and we all felt that Jessica was on her way to recovery – we had saved her leg at least for now.

When Jessica returned home, she saw a physical therapy table in the middle of her living room. The husband of one of her salon clients, Mike, stood next to it.

"I built this for you, Jessica," he said proudly.

"Mike, you shouldn't have!" said Jessica, tears forming in her eyes.

"I've built a lot of tables like this for work at the gymnasium. I know how important your physical therapy is for your recovery."

Jessica told her friends and family that she remained extremely susceptible to infections in her left leg. During the accident, skin in her heel had been totally ripped off. Although it was stitched back on, the skin never healed completely. A large crack ran down her heel as a reminder of her vulnerability – her very own Achilles' heel. A home health nurse came to Jessica's house to treat her with antibiotic injections and to draw blood to test for infections. Jessica knew that with such a high risk of infection, there was a possibility that she would have to have her lower left leg amputated. I had told her she needed to take advantage of the time that she had to rehabilitate her leg, just in case she would later lose the support of the lower half due to an amputation.

Without fail, Jessica devoted six hours a day, seven days a week, to physical therapy at home. Using her new table, she practiced standing on her leg and slowly built strength in her muscles, which had been unused for months. With all of the outpouring of love and support from churches, Jessica was able to keep her mind busy. When she was finished with her daily physical therapy, she would write down the name of everyone who had offered to help her. Before she went to bed, she logged her physical therapy hours and her progress in a journal. When she couldn't sleep, she continued to write about her experiences in that journal.

Most of the time, she struggled to share the darkest moments of her traumatic experience which were always intertwined with her faith. But when she wrote late at night, the words would flow unrelentingly. She was able to write about her pain, her loneliness, and feeling disconnected and alone in her marriage. Before long, Jessica had filled stacks of journals with her most intimate feelings. When she woke in the mornings, she was adamant to only surround herself with happy and encouraging thoughts before she began another day of physical therapy. Within a few months her hard work paid off and she was able to walk wearing a boot. Several months after that, she was walking without any help.

Jessica was over the moon about her recovery. She knew that with God's watchful gaze, she could accomplish anything. The only battles that seemed to be out of her control were the ongoing fights with Dave. Despite Jessica's positive perspective on her injury, Dave couldn't handle the changes that the accident had brought into their life

"Why isn't this working?" Dave cried with exasperation one day after a bitter fight.

Jessica's eyes became misty. She spoke openly about what Dave had been thinking this entire time. "Maybe it's easier to rebuild a broken body than a broken relationship."

They both stood in silence. A few weeks later, nearly a year after the accident, Dave filed for divorce.

Although it was something they both had felt would eventually take place, Jessica was heart-broken, but she couldn't be angry at Dave. If God could help her get through a near-death experience, He would help her with the divorce as well. Jessica couldn't bear being in the empty house by herself so she decided to stay with her childhood friend, Candace who welcomed her with open arms.

Candace lived in Florida, eleven hours away from Tennessee. At Candace's house, away from the tensions in her own home, Jessica finally felt that her mind and spirit were beginning to recover along with her body. As devastating as it was to realize that she would now have to face all of her challenges as a divorced woman, she felt at peace knowing that her life was moving forward.

When Jessica woke one morning, she felt an excruciating pain in her left leg. She wailed loudly, completely immobilized by the pain. Candace ran to Jessica's room.

"What's wrong?!" Candace cried.

"My leg," Jessica managed to say between gasps. "We need to get to Vanderbilt."

Within minutes, Jessica and Candace were in the car on their way back to Tennessee from Candace's house.

The drive back was the longest eleven hours of Jessica's life. Without any medication on hand, Jessica had nauseating pain. When Jessica came into my clinic to see me, I knew something was wrong and the moment I saw her leg, my heart sank. I looked up into Jessica's eyes. I could tell by her face that she already knew what I was going to say. She smiled and held my hand, her eyes welling up with tears. "Whatever it is, it's going to be okay." We both looked at each other and knew what had to be done – Jessica needed an amputation. We had tried everything. This moment was another demonstration of the strength that emanated from Jessica. I was two years into my practice and had done multiple surgeries to save her leg, I was invested and my heart was broken for her and she could tell. In this moment she could have done anything, yelled in anger or cried in frustration. Instead, she took my hand in hers and looked into my eyes and said, "You did everything you could and everything right, this is God's will and it's time for me to move forward.

"It's okay," she reassured me again, smiling brightly as a single tear fell down her cheek. "We'll make it through this."

In a moment of such profound loss she wasn't even thinking about herself. As I drove home that night I kept thinking about our discussion. My mind drifted back to Hillsboro and the community that always pushed forward no matter what the obstacles; that's exactly what Jessica was doing. I thought about my dad and what he would have done and what he would have said to Jessica. I thought about the case over and over again, did I do the right things? Could I have done anything different to save her leg?

The next day I took Jessica to the operating room and we found infection all through her leg. We agreed before going to surgery that we would not make any major decisions and that it would be exploratory. After surgery as I had done from the beginning I went to Jessica's bedside and gave her a hug and explained what I had found. Telling Jessica that we had no more options was one of the hardest things I have had to ever do.

Jessica thought of her friend Mark who was in a motorcycle accident thirteen years earlier. For the last decade of his life, he had undergone more than twenty surgeries trying to fight infections in his leg. Jessica knew that she didn't want to live her life that way. Rather than always be in a permanent state of recovery, Jessica wanted to be recovered. "I'm ready to have it come off," she said with determination.

After she was prepared for surgery, I brought Jessica in to the operating room. With a heavy heart, I began the procedure of amputating her leg. A few hours later, I watched as she was wheeled away. I wondered how she would feel when she saw her below knee amputation for the first time. Miraculously, when Jessica woke up and looked down at what remained of her left leg, she smiled. "I'll call it Shorty," she said.

By the time Jessica went back to her home in Franklin a few days later, she had realized that everything in her life had or would shortly be changed. She was fitted for prosthetics several times, but none of them could ever replace the true sensation of standing on her own two legs. From getting dressed in the morning to making lunch to going to the supermarket a few blocks away, nothing was the same. The drastic changes to her body drained her mind and spirit. Jessica knew that if she tried to repress the overwhelming emotions that she was feeling, she would never be able to completely recover.

Despite the setback of her amputation Jessica continued to move forward and bought her own Salon. Going to work at the salon every day was a challenge, but Jessica was determined to be a fighter. Her friends at work had been so supportive throughout this time helping in her absence, but she wanted to be able to take care of herself. She didn't want to depend on the system or anyone other than God. Every morning when she got out of bed, her legs were throbbing, screaming for her to get back to bed. Now that she and Dave were divorced, Jessica spent most of her time at home alone. Going to work gave her the chance to see other people who would lift her spirits with their love and care.

Jessica's positive attitude was an inspiration. I asked her to come and share her story with the medical students I was teaching. She immediately said yes. During the first day of my first course, I had Jessica sit with me in the front of the class. She sat in her wheelchair, beaming up at the students.

I began the class with pictures of Jessica's x-rays. The students gasped when they saw them. I explained the medical history behind Jessica's trauma before I asked for her to share her experiences. My students were mesmerized by her strength and spirit. When she finished, I turned to Jessica and finally asked her the question that I wanted to know the answer to this whole time. "How were you able to stay so upbeat, so positive? What allowed you to just keep going?"

Jessica smiled. Without saying anything, she pointed her finger up.

Speaking in my classroom was a cathartic experience for Jessica. She told me that it felt like a heavy weight had been lifted off her shoulders. Jessica's faith remained unwavering during the next few months of her recovery.

After several prosthetic fittings, the right one was found and Jessica was finally able to stand up and walk. When she first stood up on her new leg, it was a great shock to her system. The pain that would shoot up her phantom left leg at times made the entire experience surreal. The prosthetic was a reminder that her leg was truly not there, and would never be. Even worse, her right leg began having severe pain. Still, Jessica refused to take pain medications. She wanted to be able to feel the pain so that she would know when something was wrong. When the pain in her right leg became unbearable she finally came to see me. I told her that she was developing arthritis in the right knee given that she had not been placing any weight on the left side for a long time and that down the road she might need a knee replacement. In front of me as she always did she took this news in stride.

But Jessica left the clinic as if in a trance. She didn't know how she got down four floors to her car, but when she sat in the driver's seat and looked at her reflection in the mirror, she saw that her eyes were blood red. She touched her face. It was dry, and her makeup was not running. She looked down at her lap. It was filled with tears.

Jessica realized she had just hung her head and cried. Tears began streaming down her face. For the first time, Jessica became enraged with anger. The weight of everything that had happened to her during the last two years was just too much at that moment. It was all just so unfair, she felt.

Jessica was mad at the other driver, mad that her legs weren't working, mad that one of them had to be taken. Most of all, she was mad at her ex-husband for divorcing her while she was going through this horrific time. He was supposed to be her person. Everybody in life has that person, and he was hers. She fumbled in her purse and pulled out her phone. She scrolled through her list of contacts. She had three dozen close friends on speed dial who she knew would move heaven and Earth to help her. But when she looked at that list, there was not one single person she wanted to call.

Jessica continued to sob uncontrollably. Sitting in the dark garage in her car, Jessica had never felt so alone. She felt there was only one being at her side at that moment, and that was God.

"God," Jessica said in between sobs, "I need your help."

Jessica poured her heart and soul out to God. For an hour she sat there and openly spoke of everything she hadn't said aloud during the previous two years. As she espoused her feelings, she began to feel better. She felt herself surrounded by the Holy Spirit. In that moment, she realized everything would be okay.

For the next several months, Jessica's story continued to spread from one church to another. Before her next surgery, Jessica began receiving an outpouring of messages from across the community. Churches, support groups, and schools were reaching out to Jessica asking her to give motivational speeches to their community. Jessica thought back to the moment when she had talked to my group of students. She had pages and pages of stories that she wanted to share. Instead of keeping them confined within the journals in her bedroom, she realized she should share them to help inspire others. Her trauma wasn't a scar she needed to hide; it was a representation of the hardships that God had walked her through. Since she had sat in His lap on that fateful day, she knew that she would forever remain within His arms.

Jessica began speaking at events across Tennessee. Strangers began approaching Jessica on the street. "Are you Jessica Rutledge?" They would ask. Many of them wanted to share their encouragement and sympathy. Others wanted to tell her their stories and receive her guidance.

Within a few months, Jessica was speaking in large arenas before hundreds of people. When she'd look out at the crowds, at the interested people in the audience, she began to realize that maybe this was God's purpose all along.

When Jessica sat with Jansen the day before her next surgery, she tried to explain the overwhelming feelings she had felt during the last two years. "I feel as if God had taken me to the edge of a cliff," she began, gazing off into the distance. "A cliff where the only direction I could go was forward. I knew that when I stepped ahead of myself, God would either catch me or give me wings to soar. Maybe God gave me these experiences so that I could share them with others."

"I think so," agreed Jansen. "There's always a reason for everything. When you get to heaven you'll find out what it's all about," she said with a smile. Jessica smiled back. "I know I will. I already have one foot through the door."

From the day of her injury Jessica faced so many challenges that would have driven many to give up hope and quit. But Jessica continued to live a full life and push forward with the power of her faith and the devotion of her family and community. From what could have been a life ending tragedy she did not falter but instead found her voice.

Progress Notes on Jessica

Jessica has continued the long process of recovery with the help of her faith, friends, and family. She continues to do motivational speaking. She has even modified a teddy bear with a prosthetic and a crutch to educate young children about a life as an amputee. While Jessica longs to share life's journey with someone special, she's making great use of her free time writing her inspirational autobiography – "One Foot in Heaven."

EPILOGUE

During the past three years while writing this book, I have been blessed to see each of these eight patients move forward with their lives in the face of catastrophe and major adversity. Spending time with each of my patients on this project has made it clear to me that every human being has a story to tell and to truly help your patients, you must know this narrative.

Every day I remain awe struck by the power of faith, family, and community to do the impossible and heal where medicine and surgery simply cannot. As I write this, it is Fall 2015 and I'm in my fifth year as an orthopedic trauma surgeon at Vanderbilt. As I rush patients to the operating room in the face of tragedy, I often think about the stories I share here, and how far my patients must travel from sickness to reach health. But I steadfastly believe that through the power of God, the love of family, and the support of community each individual will make it through to see a brighter day. I strongly feel there is no greater privilege than to take this journey and travel this long and winding road together with my patients.

Being at home in Tennessee, I have continued the path that my mother and father started decades ago to make a difference in the lives of the communities that did so much for our family. Our non-profit organization, Healthy Tennessee, continues to grow and gain support in encouraging all Tennesseans to live a healthy lifestyle. As I have traveled across the state seeing patients and organizing health fairs, I have seen firsthand the power of Tennesseans to come together to help one another in times of need. Our youth violence prevention initiative also continues to expand and has now been introduced into the Memphis school system where we have seen encouraging results.

I often think of my father and all that he taught me and the tremendous struggles that he and my mother overcame so I could live the American Dream. Recently I had the opportunity to travel to Haiti on a medical mission trip. As I stood in a small run down three room shack in the 100-degree weather, it occurred to me that my parents had faced similar circumstances but risked it all and traveled to America and ultimately Hillsboro, Tennessee, so their children would never know the shackles of poverty that bound them.

As I watch my son and daughter grow, I am reminded of the life lessons I learned growing up in Hillsboro and the small community that loved, raised, and believed in me – it truly is the American Dream in Tennessee. Who could have imagined that the same powerful forces of faith, family, and community that propelled me forward, would be central in the recovery of my patients; it is this glue that binds us all together.

ACKNOWLEDGMENTS

I want to first and foremost thank the love of my life, Maya, for all her support and encouragement throughout this project. To my patients who opened their hearts and homes to me, I am eternally grateful for all that you have taught me. Bob Davis, a true man of faith, thank you for your unwavering support in all stages of writing this book. Rachel Thakore, I am truly grateful for your help in the initial stages of writing. Ben Keeling, Bre Mastrodonato, and Christian Hidalgo: thank you for the wonderful pictures you have taken of my family. Finally, Tim O'Brien, thank you for believing in this project and helping me find my voice.

ACKNOWLEDGMENTS

[illegible]

About the author
MANNY SETHI, M.D.

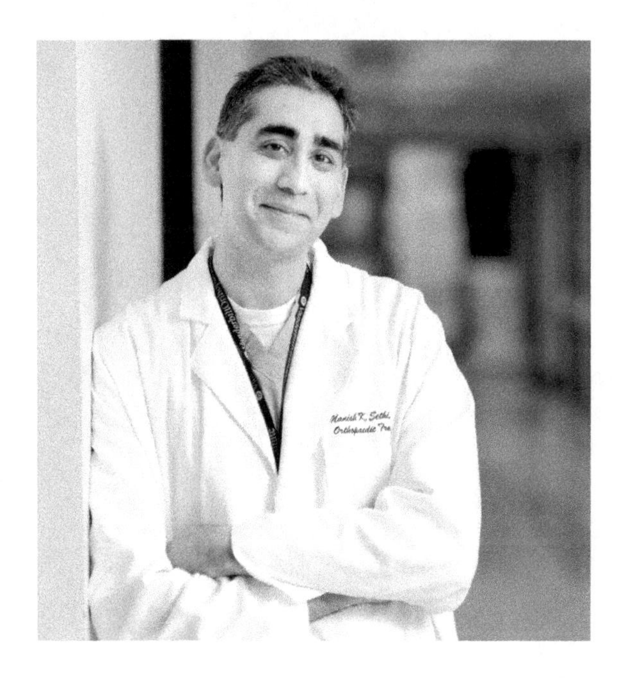

Manny Sethi is an Orthopedic Trauma surgeon at Vanderbilt University Medical Center and was raised in Hillsboro, Tennessee, where his mother and father practiced medicine for over 20 years. Dr. Manny is also the president and founder of Healthy Tennessee, a non-profit organization dedicated to preventative health education across the state. He is married to his high school sweetheart Maya, and together they have two children.